QUANTUM BRAIN HEALING

Dr. Rebecca Bell Stone, MD India

The author of this book holds a Medical Degree in Alternative Medicine and a Masters Degree in Oriental Medicine. The purpose of this book is to advise you on healthcare options available for several diseases and conditions in the brain. It does not remove the requirement for you to seek the supervision of your regular physician or medical provider. The author expressly disclaims responsibility for the adverse effect arising from the use of any treatment or application found in this book. No treatment or plan works for every person and the physician administering the treatment may not follow the protocol shown in the book. Each person's body chemistry is different.

This book is intended to provide help in delaying the onset or progression of many brain diseases and conditions. It also offers suggestions on how to improve your brain function and increase your ability to function at a higher level.

Book Dedication

This book is dedicated to my mentors, doctors, deans, and teachers: Dr. Y. Omura; Dr. Devi Namibudred; Mala and Mohan; Dr. Daniel Kirsch; Dr. Mu; Dr. Terry Rives, PhD; Dr. Lisa Lin of TCTCM in Austin; Dr. Guili Zheng; Dr. Baisong Zhong; Dr K. Liu; Dr. Wen; the great Dr. Heidi Seifert of Seifert Pain Clinic in Houston; Dr. Dong; Dr. M. Groves; Dr. Frank Chen; Louis Chen LAc; Dr. Ken Mathis; Dr. Bruce Smith; Dr. Ron Walters; Dr. Thomas Wang; Dr. Kuo; Shirley Brown; Lois McConnell; Dr. Craig Williams; Dr. Shen Ping Liang; John Paul Liang, LAc; Minmai Liang; Mr. Diaz; Donna Brazile; Principal Robert Smith; Dean Ho; UT President William Powers; Art instructor Lois Abrom; Dr. Guo; Dr. Tom Anderson; Dean McMillan; Dr. Thomas Granchi; Dr. Chuck Brunacardi; Dr. Marvin Lerner; Dr. Woods; Dr. Geoffrey Steinbauer; Dr. Bob Marshall; William Faloon; Life Extension Foundation; Dr. Honora Wolfe; Dr. Mark Katz; Dr. Jessica Liu; Mary Helen and John Fason; Magdi; William Morris, LAc of AOMA in Austin; Marilyn Allen, LAc; the late Dr. DeBakey; A4M; ICAET; and Dr. Melinda Superville.

My family, including the late Drs. Neal and Franklin Owens, my grandmother Professor Bell Owens Livingston, Gone Daddy, Rupert Scott, Frank Scott, my grandparents Dorothy Pat Scott and James Embry Stone, Bebe Penney, my parents Marguerite and Scott Stone, Loretta Bonner, Elaine, Charles and Jo Ann Schooley, Susan Rose Stone Taborn, Kitty Owens, Annabelle Taborn, Jackie Stone, Tiffany Stone, Michael Stone Taborn, John Trombly, Mary Mathis, John Mathis, Bill and Judith Moyers, Bill and Suzanne, Sammy, Marianne and Steve, Majorie Love, Mark and Julie, Mary Jane Love, the Landry family, Jimmy and Caroline Parsons, Linda and Bill Raman, Lynette and M.C., Howard, Royal Family of Scotland, the House of Orange, and the Medici family.

I want to thank Claudio Parrini for his great art that I adore and is on the cover of the book. KUDOS to Roy Francis for a wonderful job and I will always appreciate his help on my book. Thanks to Travis Crane for his early assistance when I needed it! The fabulous attorneys of Ross and Mathews: Brian Ross, Mary Hardy and Diane Kelly. Better than you have a right to expect or demand!

My people and places that have inspired me along the way, including Clark Smith, Rick Vicens, Rai Barghava, Mark Laufman, Joe Roberts, Glen Kinder, Ghopal Rana, Bob Fagan, Mike Morris, Clint Fawcett, Murray, Truman, Joey, Gene, Tom Devins, K.C.Weiner, Rusty, Anita Stovall, Art Swanson, Ed Ritterhouse (thanks!!), Ken Randolph, Carson, Charles Cusack, Chris Terry, Chris, Bill Stavinoha, Bill Damon, Bill Griffin, Ron Cochran, Mary Bowers and her family, Tensley, Rayma, my big sister Susan Pontello, Brenda Petty, Steve Hartzelle, Susan Dunnaway, Walter Hurt, Bobby Mims, David Towner, Jim Martin, Daryl, Don Smith, Ron Ross, Coralie Sculley, Roilyn Lentz, Dora Thomas, Buddy Bell, Lt. Gov. David Dewhurst, Greg Abbott, the Pecore family, Ann Zimmerer, Rod Miller (thanks!), Marianne and Tim White, the Natalie and Alexis Jacobs family, the Chase Family, the Bonhams, Steve Windell, Tom Rommel, Connie Carlile, my favorite CEO Al Glancy, the talented John Bryson, Bob Edgell, Jim Iaco (thanks!), Scott and Nancy, Kevin McCracken, Kevin Fox, Chuck Davario, the Enron jedi, Robert Paladino, Greg Bafalis, Diana Spencer, Joan Carter, Julia Richardson, Dominique and John De Menil, Robert Riley, the great Jim Pignatelli, the late Romano Salvatori, Ted Baldwin, Glen Smith (thanks!), Rick Blanford, Bill Klesse, Bob Mead (thanks!), Archie Jacoby, Bob, Tammy Dewhurst, Lily, Pat and Charlie Ricker, Dr. Nancy Anderson, Erik Anderson's Sacred Lands, Queen Elizabeth, the Henry Plant Museum in Tampa, St. Petersburg Sunken Gardens, the Menil Museum, Carlos Slim, Vincente Fox, the Henry Parritius, Rothko Chapel, Ava Maria Grotto, St. John Vianney Church, Reverend Bell of St. Austins Church (thanks!), Dr. David de Jongh, Mike Parks, Kathy Kinnon, Howard and Katherine Acton, Daryl Hartnett, the Kunsthaus, ABB, the Jim McCain family, Don Smith, Suzanne Rowell, Jerry Bruner, Miles Allen, Sacred Heart Cathedral, Sister Virginia O'Donnell, Sandy Hobbs, Melinda Brown, Yuli, Doug Shows, the Art League of Alexandria, the Austin Art Alliance, Judy Jaffe, Toy Mitchell, Mark Bauer, Allen Stoner, Nancy Stoner, Beth

Stoner, Mitchy Howell, Tim Howe (thanks!), my dear friend Near and Far, the Austin Film Festival, Lance, Andrew, and my late friend Robert Chaney.

Table of Contents

INTRODUCTION

Quantum Brain Healing has been developed after many years of research. It is a blend of Orthomolecular Medicine, Traditional Chinese Medicine, Ayurvedic herbs, laser therapy, Nambudripad's Allergy Elimination Techniques (NAET), far infrared therapy, food therapy, neurofeedback, behavioral modification therapies, Amino Acid Therapy, or Bach Flower Remedies, combined with a wide variety of additional alternative concepts. At least eighty alternative therapies have been reviewed and utilized to expand the healing of the most serious brain conditions and symptoms.

It is our goal to take the best and most progressive therapies available and combine them in a manner that enhances or expands the use and effectiveness of all forms of alternative medicine. This form of alternative medicine may be the most affordable type of medicine for the many citizens without insurance – this area of medicine will grow in importance due to the lack of insurance for the masses. It is a non-invasive and non-painful type of medicine. Alternative medicine usually has few side effects, but there are occasionally allergic reactions to dietary changes, herbs, and nutritional supplements.

Quantum Brain Healing enhances brain quality and function through the use of Orthomolecular Medicine and alternative medicine therapies to treat and heal many brain diseases and reduce brain symptoms. It uses therapeutic doses of amino acids, vitamins, minerals, herbs, botanical extracts, and nutritional products to change brain chemistry and heal the brain without drugs. It can reduce the levels of drugs that have many side effects or replace drugs for those who fail to respond to them.

The protocols outlined in Quantum Brain Healing may require several months or several years, depending upon the length of time the person has had his disease or symptom. It is also extremely important to recognize that many brain symptoms mimic a brain disease, and diagnostic testing results may not confirm the expected diagnosis. These symptoms can often be cleared up with early treatment and alternative medicine therapies. Remove the environmental factors that are associated with your disease to improve your outcome. Research your family tree for undiagnosed brain symptoms or diseases and exercise extreme care if people in your family suffer from drug, nicotine, or alcohol addiction. Avoid tobacco, alcohol, and recreational drugs when addiction history is present. These addictions are usually due to genetic weaknesses that worsen during stress or life-changing events, such as divorce, death, or bankruptcy. Many brain symptoms can be delayed or avoided if proactive diet and exercise changes are incorporated into your life.

There is an explosion of brain disease. Children are developing attention deficit disorder

(ADD), autism, genetic disorders, type 1 diabetes, learning disabilities, and attention deficit hyperactivity disorder (ADHD) at ever-accelerating rates, with very little explanation of the genetic changes that allow more brain diseases to strike people at younger ages. Adults are suffering from Alzheimer's, type 2 diabetes, memory loss, brain fog, panic disorder, and multiple sclerosis at younger ages. Many times a doctor is unable to diagnose the diseases due to the wide range of the patient's symptoms. Patients often react to brain symptoms and disorders by increasing their intake of sugar, caffeine, nicotine, drugs, alcohol, and over-the-counter drugs. This also makes their diagnoses challenging for any type of health care provider.

Long-term dietary and lifestyle changes have resulted in drastic increases in drug addiction, alcohol abuse, nicotine addiction, and eating disorders. Increased use of pesticides and chemical fertilizers can lead to early Alzheimer's disease, cognitive disorders, and poor memory. Refined foods, food dyes, food additives, and genetically modified foods have resulted in the need for most people to take nutritional supplements to achieve adequate nutrition. The produce available now has lower levels of vitamins and minerals.

Many therapies will not work or are not needed for everyone who suffers from a specific brain condition. The options are wide and varied; patients with improper diagnoses or undiagnosed brain symptoms have options to pursue. Some important concepts will not be discussed here concerning the delivery mechanisms for certain supplements to pass the blood-brain barrier because such medical options are understood only by those with medical training. Quantum Brain Healing seeks to provide alternative medical options for improved brain health, but it does not provide medical training.

There is a suggested order and scope for these healing therapies. Quantum Brain Healing focuses on affordable brain healing and making life changes that enable the patients to retain the improvement in their health and prevent symptoms from returning. There are often opportunities to heal the body and brain after brain symptoms have surfaced but before the onset of the full disease. It is these cases we hope to prevent from manifesting into serious brain diseases.

Eating on the run and the high divorce rate are two common reasons for a disruption in mealtimes. Many families no longer eat breakfast together at the table. Children eat a Pop-Tart or bagel while riding in a carpool or on the bus to school. Children's diets are very high in refined sugar and carbohydrates.

The wide scope of chemicals, air pollution, pesticides, food dyes, food additives, water pollutants, electromagnetic pollution, computer radiation, and cell phone radiation has contributed to the genesis of many new illnesses; there also are more cases of existing illnesses and frequently, these may manifest in young children or teenagers. Detoxification is a key element in dealing with these many health issues, including most brain illnesses.

For years, alternative health-care practitioners have recommended using nutritional supplementation due to the decline in mineral content in the soil. The poor mineral content, along with pesticides and air pollution, has resulted in produce that delivers fewer health benefits. Vitamin and mineral supplements must be taken in order to get an adequate amount of nutrients on a daily basis and this is true even for a person without a major illness. Therapeutic levels of vitamins, minerals, and nutritional supplements also are needed by those who experience diminished brain function, impaired memory, weakened concentration, or attention deficits.

Quantum Brain Healing is able to heal or improve many brain illnesses, including ADD, addiction, ADHD, Alzheimer's disease, amnesia, anxiety, Asperser's syndrome, auditory hallucinations, autism, bipolar disorder, depression, cognitive disorders, concentration problems, dyslexia, eating disorders, epilepsy, forgetfulness, ischemia, mania, migraine headaches, multiple sclerosis, neuropathy, panic disorder, Parkinson's disease, post-traumatic stress disorder (PTSD), obsessive-compulsive disorder (OCD), seizure disorder, stress disorder, and stroke.

Good brain function relies on positive inputs into the body as well as the removal of negative inputs such as nicotine, excess alcohol, over-the-counter medications, unnecessary prescription drugs, addictive foods, and recreational drugs. Your healthy brain requires that the harmful elements of your life be removed or reduced and replaced with healthy diets, exercise, relaxation techniques, nutritional supplements, food-based vitamins, and alternative therapies.

Quantum Brain Healing believes that your brain is influenced by many factors, including your work, your physical environment, the food and beverages you consume, and the people with whom you are interact on a daily basis. The physical environment may be laden with toxins that are impossible to avoid, such as electromagnetic toxins, and those that you can manage, such as cell phones. The television and movies that you include in your life are a type of programming for your mind and can improve or impair your brain function. Newspapers, magazines, and books can stimulate and increase your brain health. Card and computer games will stimulate brain function. Doing research on the Internet can enhance your neural network and improve your mental function. It is very important for children as well as the elderly to focus on ways to increase their IQ or brain activity.

You can increase your intelligence and brain function by the choices you make, which can enhance the brain's energetic flow to increase or expand intelligence. It is always important to choose health care professionals that have goals similar to yours. Interview your health care professional to ensure that you are on the same page. A health care provider should share your vision and desired outcome for a healthy life. Movies, reading materials, television, exercise, and music can affect your brain and its performance.

Quantum Brain Healing understands that there are often simple explanations for brain symptoms like brain fog, poor memory, concentration problems, and cognitive disorders. For example, it may be a hormone problem. Hormone problems can occur in young and old alike. Often, high levels of plastic toxins alter and affect the body in a way similar to estrogen. Children can experience strange symptoms including growing breasts or having excess adipose tissue beyond that due to poor eating habits due to hormone problems; middle-aged people are susceptible to hormone deficiencies. Enzymatic Therapy sells porcine thyroid glandular supplements that can improve memory, concentration, and intelligence in people with low or borderline thyroid levels.

Thyroid deficiency symptoms include hair loss, constipation, weight gain, susceptibility to infections and illness, skin infections, brittle nails, depression, memory lapses, concentration problems, irritability, fatigue, low energy, dry or cracked skin, cold intolerance, anxiety, thinning of the outer eyebrows, excessive sleep, low body temperature, low sex drive, chronic sinus infections, and menstrual problems.

Successful supplementation should be carefully monitored with frequent basal temperature monitoring or blood tests. Supplements from animals raised on organic or chemical-free farms are best. Synthetic thyroid does not work for everyone; glandular supplements can be a good option. Bio-identical hormones can be obtained to replace several hormone deficiencies that negatively affect brain function.

Long-term deficiency of omega-3 and omega-6 fatty acids can seriously impair concentration, learning, memory, and neural plasticity. Neurotransmitter and amino acid deficiencies also will result in impaired memory and intelligence. Good food choices should be the base platform, and nutritional supplements should be added to provide therapeutic benefit for those with brain symptoms and problems. Orthomolecular Medicine can include Amino Acid Therapy and botanical herbal extracts to treat problems with fluctuating moods and metal clarity.

Brain inflammation can cause poor memory, concentration problems, and delays in word recall. It is important to avoid sugar-laden foods that create significant inflammation in the brain and throughout the body. Chemical additives in water and food should also be avoided. Pure filtered or mineral spring water is a good idea, since dehydration is one of the chief ways that the brain becomes sluggish. Alcohol can destroy brain cells and should be avoided in excess. Foods that are extremely high in antioxidants are good neuroprotectants.

Many foods can enhance the brain by increasing clarity, memory, and intelligence; some foods have chemical properties that can protect and enhance brain function. These foods are açai berry extract, blueberries, blackberries, raspberries, cherries, prunes, strawberries, raisins, red grapes, plums, kale, spinach, brussels sprouts, walnuts, almonds, flaxseed, whey protein, eggs, garlic, leeks, cold-water fish, organic coffee, and organic tea. Foods that can impair brain function include alcohol, carbonated beverages, juices that are high in sugar, MSG, food dyes, sugar substitutes, nitrates, refined foods, and foods that are charred or very well done. It is very important to always eat breakfast to maintain good brain function. A late afternoon snack with protein can also improve your energy and brain function.

Quantum Brain Healing expands its concept of healing to environmental choices that the patient makes on a daily basis. Electromagnetic toxins and radiation must be kept to a minimum. Each person needs to make choices concerning level of cell phone radiation, wireless Internet system overlaps and frequency settings, home wireless telephone systems for the home, and proximity to high-voltage electric power lines. Broadband and fiber optics are good choices in today's environment for phone, television, and Internet choices. Wireless technologies impact your body's neurological system. Limit wireless technology when designing the interior of your home. Your body will have better hormone and neurotransmitter regulation when there is less stimulation at night in your sleeping environment.

Design your home to minimize noise pollution if you live in a metropolitan area. Make your new cell phone purchases after researching the level of cell phone radiation for the new phone models. It is also wise to purchase a device for your cell phone that reduces cell phone radiation it can be purchased at many locations online, including Amazon. Eliminate electric blankets and electrical devices near the bed.

Place all electrical devices as far away from your head as possible in your bedroom. This will help reduce electromagnetic pollution and the interruption of your circadian rhythm. The body's production of hormones is affected by the circadian rhythm. This disruption may cause declining production of melatonin, L-dopa, serotonin, and DHEA. Hormone regulation and balance is key to optimal brain function. Careful monitoring of hormone levels during midlife is very important to maintaining a balanced and problem-free brain. Quantum Brain Healing believes that bio-identical hormones, Chinese herbal formulas, and Amino Acid Therapy are the best alternative health-care choices to correct hormone deficiencies.

ADDICTIONS

Quantum Brain Healing utilizes many therapies for dealing with addiction, including Amino Acid Therapy, therapeutic vitamins and minerals, acupuncture, laser therapy, Emotional Freedom Technique (EFT), and herbal formulas. Detoxification is needed before nutritional therapies are used for most people. Vaccines are on the horizon that may help many with substance abuse. The Cambridge University-based Xenova Group PLC is developing therapeutic vaccines for cocaine and nicotine addiction.

Addiction vaccines are designed to prime the immune system to produce anti-cocaine or anti-nicotine antibodies. The addictive substance binds to the antibodies after entering the bloodstream. The resulting large antibody complex cannot cross the blood-brain barrier, so the usually pleasurable stimulus is absent or reduced. These vaccines will help those who wish to stop using cocaine or nicotine; the vaccines also may be used to prevent addiction. If clinical trials are successful, such a vaccine should seriously be considered in families where there is significant history of addiction.

When attempting substance abuse withdrawal, the use of amino acid supplements is key to stabilizing the brain's neurological function when it is attacked by addiction stressors such as drugs, alcohol, shopping, computer, pornography, and sex. The removal of the addiction stressors cannot be achieved without severe destabilization of key brain functions. People of certain DNA types are predisposed to substance abuse problems. Look to your family history to determine these issues. Dual addictions are common in families with a history of addiction disorders. Drugs and alcohol or cigarettes and alcohol are common dual addictions. Examine the onset of the addiction relative to events that occurred around the time of onset, and discuss these issues with your doctor. Chinese medicine incorporates the emotional factors into the treatment.

Chemical support through pharmacology, herbs, nutritional supplements, amino acids, minerals, vitamins, or nootropics will produce improved withdrawal outcomes and better long-term remission rates. The hormone and neurotransmitters need to be supported. The hypothalamic-pituitary-adrenal (HPA) axis will be drastically affected as neuroendocrine levels rise or fall. Chinese herbs have many chemical components and can act quickly in the body or brain when the right herb is selected.

Morphine, heroin, and other opiate molecules can occupy receptor sites on the GABA-releasing neurons ordinarily reserved for endorphins, creating an accentuated high. For patients who are in morphine or other opiate withdrawal, Quantum Brain Healing introduces the herb Rhodiola rosea to activate the opioid receptors. This will reduce some of the stress associated with opiate withdrawal for most patients (those who are not allergic to the herb).

Quantum Brain Healing will add the amino acid supplement GABA for a smoother drug detoxification process during the one-month withdrawal period. Nootropics are drugs or other nutritional products that can increase your IQ and make you smarter. They are sometimes used by older people returning to law school or medical school to master higher learning after their brain has aged. Nootropic substances can aid the brain in rewiring itself with new neural pathways. Over time, the normal baseline functioning may equalize with Rhodiola, GABA, 5-HTP, and other nootropic supplements. Altering the nutrient protocol over time as the patient's brain changes is key. Life Extension nutritional products are a great way to achieve these brain enhancements.

An addicted brain has damaged neurons and signaling functions that require time to heal and need biochemical support. Micropolarity will be altered. The old neural paths are damaged and degraded with significant drug abuse. Nootropic substances are needed to create new neural pathways and repair DNA damage.

Brahmi is an Ayurvedic herb that improves protein synthesis in brain-cell repair and encourages new neuron growth. The suggested course of action is to implement scalp and auricular (ear) acupuncture with herbs and amino acids to stimulate new nerve growth. The acupuncture will help facilitate new neural networks; it may work more quickly if electro-acupuncture is used. (This treatment is common for most acupuncturists.) The patient should be able to notice a significant difference within ten to twenty electro-acupuncture treatments if there is no relapse in substance abuse. Brain waves should normalize somewhat during this treatment period.

Dopamine-producing nerve cells in the mid-brain are a possible future target to prevent relapses of drug dependence. Dopamine-producing nerve cells are central to the brain's reward system and become more excitable when a person takes drugs. Dopamine is involved in appetite, sex, motivation, and aggression. Dopamine imbalances may cause situations in which there is an inability to derive pleasure from a normally happy situation. Complex thinking, emotions, and moods are affected by dopamine, serotonin, and noradrenaline.

Quantum Brain Healing uses herbs such as Rhodiola, deer antler, horny goat weed, dan shen, black cohosh, yohimbe, and ginseng to stimulate the production of dopamine and help balance the brain. CoQ10 and fish oil also can increase brain levels of dopamine and serotonin. Orthomolecular Amino Acid Therapy also may be used when needed. Long-term therapeutic use of amino acids, vitamins, minerals, and herbs will be needed for some people with long-term addictions or family predispositions.

Cocaine increases the number of glutamate receptors in a person, making the neuron more excitable. Blocking this increase of receptor sites helps prevent relapses into addiction.

Stimulating the region of the brain that contains the neurotransmitter glutamate, however, causes a relapse of cocaine addiction. Using Quantum Molecular Medicine to stimulate dopamine in the brain has an anti-aging effect and increases brain plasticity. Anything with the ability to increase your brain's plasticity can increase IQ, if properly done. This could be important for people with long-term drug and alcohol abuse problems because the abuse causes significant brain cell death. Rebuilding and rewiring the brain is essential for drug abusers and addicts. Most eating addictions can be healed with Amino Acid Therapy and nutritional support, along with psychotherapy. Addictions stemming from sexual abuse will be more difficult to treat. Treating any patient while he or she is being abused, sexually or physically, remains challenging.

Electrical stimulation of the hippocampus, the part of the brain involved in forming memory and organizing, with electro-acupuncture may rewire the memory-based patterns associated with long-term drug use. This could lead to an understanding that there is a hyper-polarity in the hippocampus that needs to be sedated initially to create new neural networks to alter this function. Scalp acupuncture can be used to reduce or increase the polarity. This research is documented in China.

Quantum Brain Healing Alternatives for Addiction

> Laser Therapy with Luminex or Thor Laser

> Scalp Acupuncture

> Auricular or Ear Acupuncture

> Electro-Therapy Acupuncture

> Chinese Patent Formulas

> Single Herbs

> Ayurvedic Medicine

> Botanical Extracts

> NAET

> Detoxification with Diet

> Foot Ionizing Detox

> Far Infrared Sauna Detox

> Magnet Therapy

> Yoga

> EEG Biofeedback

- Medical Qi Gong

- Qi Gong

- Orthomolecular Amino Acid Therapy

- Bach Flower Remedy

- Visualization

- Vitamin and Mineral IV Therapy

- Transcranial Magnetic Stimulation

- Hypnotherapy

- Eye Movement Desensitization and Reprocessing

- Aromatherapy

- Applied Behavior Analysis

Quantum Brain Healing also uses ear acupuncture with needles, electricity, or laser therapy for managing addiction withdrawal. Ear acupuncture, also referred to as auricular acupuncture, performed with laser therapy has the highest success rate in addiction recovery for most people. A hand-held electrical device can stimulate specific addiction points and brain points located on the ear and is fairly successful in managing addiction withdrawal and recovery for people afraid of needles. The best outcomes involved ear therapy five days per week for a month and three times per week for six months to a year afterward. This therapy, however, can be expensive and many working people do not have the financial ability to get such extremely frequent treatment. (Many of the studies that showed the effectiveness were on drug addicts in prison.)

Laser therapy works really well and should be tried where available. The laser used for addiction treatment is a Class III Medical Grade Cold Laser by Luminex or Thor Laser. Ask your medical professionals about the specifics on their laser. The pen-sized lasers and LED pens deliver too little power to work well. An exception is the carpel tunnel therapy protocol developed by Dr. Margaret Naeser of Boston University. It is also imperative to not overuse laser medicine in the immediate area of endocrine glands because this can harm the glands.

Dependence-inducing substances and recreational drugs cause concentrations of dopamine to rise in the area, which in turn affects other nerve cells and brings about various physical and mental reactions. One way to diminish the desire for drugs is to block the dopamine-producing nerve cell's glutamate receptors. Dopamine-producing nerve cells are central to the brain's reward system. This will cause cravings for cocaine to slow or stop. Herbal formulas can be used for this purpose, as can specific amino acid combinations.

Smokers with a specific gene for an enzyme that regulates dopamine in the brain have concentration problems and cognitive deficits when abstaining from nicotine. This gene affects the dopamine level in the pre-frontal cortex.

Tobacco contains over four thousand chemicals, and marijuana contains over four hundred. Dopamine is increased with most substance abuse, including cocaine, marijuana, heroin, alcohol, and nicotine. These drugs activate the reward system and cause neurons to release large amounts of dopamine. Over time, the dopamine overstimulates the brain to the point of damage, and the person requires a higher baseline level of dopamine in order to feel good. This altered neurotransmitter function impacts every activity that produces elevated moods. Drug abuse will negatively impact your sex life, your appetite, and your ability to feel pleasure or motivation for regular activities.

Smoking impacts the dopamine levels and increases glutamate-mediated transmission throughout brain-reward circuitries. Smoking is a way in which people attempt to self-medicate, and there is an increased risk of relapse when attempting to quit—some people attempt to quit multiple times before finding success. Quitting smoking can be dealt with biochemically, compensating for altered dopamine levels by supplementing with amino acids and nootropics to allow withdrawal without transferring problems to other types of addiction. Do not, for example, attempt to quit smoking and get off coffee at the same time. Switch to organic coffee. The protocol for quitting smoking may include SAM-e or 5-HTP and milk thistle. It is important to include herbs or amino acids that target the liver as well as the brain due to the buildup of toxins in the liver cause by the addictive substances. Herbs that treat drug and nicotine addiction include lobelia, passionflower, and skullcap.

Heavy-Metals Poisoning

Quantum Brain Healing understands that heavy-metals toxins are a large consequence of long-term smoking and drug use. Illegal drugs often contain toxins, as they might have been manufactured in homes and alleys. Cigarettes manufactured in factories have up to four thousand toxins added. These heavy-metals toxins must be removed from your body for you to survive. Detoxification of heavy metals also might help you to get off drugs and cigarettes more easily.

Heavy-metals poisoning creates many health problems. In addition to certain addictions that cause heavy-metals exposure, you also may be exposed to toxins in water contaminated with drugs, feces, heavy metals, or pesticides, certain foods, the atmosphere, the workplace, reclaimed soil, or vaccines, as well as at a toxic waste site or refuse disposal site. Symptoms and diseases vary for different heavy metals, but problems may include impaired memory, loss of certain cognitive skills, insomnia, depression, anxiety, food allergies, stress, attention deficit hyperactivity disorder (ADHD), obsessive-compulsive disorder (OCD), impaired digestion, neuropathy, colitis, delirium, hallucination, fatigue (or chronic fatigue), impaired concentration, brain fog, stupor, numbness, hair loss, impaired liver function, lymphoma, auditory problems, muscle weakness, learning disabilities, dementia, amyotrophic lateral sclerosis (ALS, also known as Lou Gehrig's disease), Parkinson's disease, certain types of multiple sclerosis (MS), and cancer.

Research shows that heavy metals are present in the nucleus of the many cancer cells. Some cancers may go into remission or be cured with detoxification and immune system stimulation.

The heavy metals and contaminants encountered in street drugs are always a problem for the addict and many doctors have not considered this issue when evaluating their patient's addiction health issues. We encounter heavy metals such as aluminum, mercury, lead, arsenic, copper, thallium, and titanium on a constant basis in our daily lives. These metals become more dangerous when heat is applied. One example is the aluminum pods for coffee that are heated by hot water as coffee is made. Another example is cans of food or carbonated beverages that become heated during transport or while stored in warehouses in the summer or in hot climates, such as the Middle East or any desert climate. Cooking food in older aluminum pots may transfer aluminum into the cooked food, and adding vinegar to any dish cooked in aluminum may make this worse.

Mercury poisoning can cause social withdrawal or interaction problems, depression, mood disorders, aggressive behavior, OCD, autism, insomnia, delirium, hallucinations, chronic fatigue, eating disorders, suicidal threats, ADHD, weakness, fatigue, speech problems, colitis, difficulty walking, temper tantrums, hearing loss, convulsions, seizures, birth defects, spontaneous abortion, motor problems, rashes, skin problems, nausea, vomiting, diarrhea, stomach cramps, allergies, asthma, and neurological problems.

Aluminum poisoning can cause Alzheimer's disease, fatigue or chronic fatigue, weakness, dementia, skin problems, rashes, motor disturbances, neurological problems, allergies, asthma, infertility issues, and respiratory diseases.

Lead poisoning can cause memory problems, concentration difficulty, depression, mood swings, irritability, insomnia, sleep disturbance, anxiety, eating disorders, ADHD, mental retardation, impaired intelligence, birth defects, spontaneous abortion, neurological problems, convulsions, seizures, headaches, muscle pain, hypertension, cardiac problems, and suppressed immune function.

The skin is the major organ through which our body detoxifies. Our body also filters toxins from the blood system through the liver, kidneys, gallbladder, and the lymphatic system. The kidneys may be overloaded during the detox process of heavy metals and pesticides. It is important to detoxify these systems and organs by drinking plenty of pure water. The body has a built-in mechanism to help detoxification of heavy metals—eating many raw fruits and vegetables and sweating. Most people don't produce enough sweat due to time spent using computers, TV, cars, dishwashers, and other items that reduce physical activity. Any exercise that produces sweat helps to detoxify the body. You also can reduce the heavy-metal load on the body, diet, nutritional supplements, intravenous chelation therapy, far infrared sauna, foot ionizing detoxification, and hot yoga.

Several oral chelation formulas reduce heavy metals; these can be purchased at health food stores. Beneficial nutritional supplements include cilantro, chlorella, liquid chlorophyll, Nori algae, dulse, barley, wheatgrass, alfalfa, kelp, alpha lipoic acid, L-cysteine, methionine, vitamin C, garlic, MSM, and pectin.

People who lack receptors for the chemical messenger dopamine are hyper sensitive and over-react to alcohol, cocaine, and methamphetamine. Their bodies may react to these substances similar to an allergic reaction. This is not the case, however, for those afflicted with schizophrenia.

Schizophrenics crave cocaine because of their impaired dopamine receptors that are less sensitive, and they often have elevated dopamine requirements. There is usually an altered brain metabolism rate, either faster or slower. Is their brain polarity lower due to this higher dopamine requirement going unsatisfied? Cocaine does not usually increase the amount of available dopamine. It can alter the polarity in a manner that benefits schizophrenics, or dopamine levels can be raised by adding supplemental amino acids. This should be monitored with diagnostic testing on a monthly basis until stable, then quarterly.

Herbs or herbal extracts that are used to treat alcohol addiction include kudzu, lobelia, vinpocetine, American ginseng, licorice (the root, not the candy), gotu kola, saffron, and skullcap. Herbs that treat drug and nicotine addiction include Bacopa monnieri, lobelia, mugwort, passionflower, skullcap, kava, and milk thistle.

Quantum Brain Healing also utilizes the herb skullcap for calming or sedating a part of the brain. Skullcap and Orthomolecular Medicine may be useful in speeding the balancing of neurotransmitter levels. Most brain diseases are rooted in the basis of unbalanced neurotransmitters. Amino acids can quickly rebalance the neurotransmitter levels when the correct ones are chosen and the correct ratio of amino acids is used. This is difficult to achieve for those medical professionals without experience in Orthomolecular Medicine.

Scutellaria lateriflora, or blue skullcap, has sedative, anticonvulsive, and anti-inflammatory effects on the brain.

Skullcap may be used to treat brain disease including epilepsy, ADD, insomnia, hysteria, anxiety, delirium, headaches, neuralgia, and convulsions. Skullcap can be used in addiction disorders to alleviate symptoms of withdrawal from barbiturates, alcohol, and tranquilizers. This Quantum Brain herb should be used in an overall treatment plan for those suffering from addictions.

Preventing brain disease and protecting the brain are important steps in an anti-aging program. It is possible to remove twelve to twenty biological years from your brain. This will allow you to work longer and perform complex tasks with ease.

Quantum Brain Healing uses saffron for to treat alcoholism. It can reduce the desire for food or drugs. It affects satiety levels in the brain. Saffron also prevents mutation in DNA. Saffron is used in Ayurvedic and Traditional Chinese Medicine as a stimulant and antioxidant. It inhibits platelet aggregation and helps prevent arteriosclerosis. It crosses the blood-brain barrier and increases circulation. Saffron can prevent cancer and can prevent and slow tumor formation. This herb can increase neurotransmitter levels. Saffron is one of the most expensive herbal products, but there is a very good product made by Quantum Nutritional Labs.

It is important to try to remove heavy-metals toxins before taking saffron if you are using it to prevent cancer or slow tumor growth. Some medical professionals suggest there are heavy metals in the nucleus of cancer cells. Removal of heavy metals will speed recovery in most diseases. Detoxification will increase significantly the results of most Orthomolecular Medicine treatment protocols. If you have tumor issues, please have your hormones tested and treated, along with this protocol. Hormone deficiencies are often connected to tumor formation. This is especially true for thyroid hormones.

Saffron is an antispasmodic and may help prevent irregular brain-wave activity caused by head injury and brain trauma. This antispasmodic effect might be beneficial in brain diseases characterized by tics such as Tourette's or transient tic disorder. Be careful about using saffron if you are taking blood thinners, drinking large quantities of green tea, or taking fish oil supplements due to their ability to further thin the blood.

Saffron can help treat headaches and depression that arise from insufficient blood circulation in the brain. These types of headaches and depression also may benefit from yoga and mild exercise. Saffron is useful in helping with alcoholism by reducing the desire for alcohol, but the addition of several amino acids will be necessary. Milk thistle also could be included in the protocol for the alcohol withdrawal and two additional herbs that would be replaced as the patient progressed through the treatment.

Lemon balm acts on the hippocampus area of the brain and functions as an antispasmodic. It can treat the heightened stress and anxiety associated with drug and smoking addiction. It also can treat the nervous exhaustion associated with drug withdrawal. Do not confuse lemon balm with lemongrass. Lemongrass is very good for reducing pesticides and heavy metals and has very different properties. Do not use lemon balm if you suffer from hypothyroid disease. This could create serious health care problems.

Lemon balm can help clear the brain for improve learning. Lemon balm can act as an antidepressant for mild depression. Quantum Brain Healing also uses lemon balm to treat primary brain disease or secondary brain symptoms from diseases targeting other body organs. Lemon balm is a great herb because of its strong medical properties and mildness. Quantum Brain Healing uses this herb as an antiviral and antibiotic agent. Lemon balm is a sedative and antioxidant. It can be used to treat stress, anxiety, or nervous exhaustion. This herb acts on the brain in many ways to reduce signs of aging. Aging of the brain may be accelerated by bacterial and viral infections that go undiagnosed and untreated. Any herb that has antibiotic and antiviral actions may be taken on a regular basis to prevent this type of occurrence. Severe eating disorders and smoking may accelerate onset of Alzheimer's disease; lemon balm can be used to prevent mild to moderate dementia.

Lobelia is a great herb that crosses the blood-brain barrier and increases norepinephrine release from the hippocampus. It stimulates the release of dopamine, has a sedating effect, and is an anxiolytic (relieves anxiety). It can increase cognitive performance. It may be useful in treating drug withdrawal symptoms, smoking cessation, depression, and headaches. It may also be useful in treating overall inflammation, such as arthritic conditions. It helps with the hyperactivity of ADHD and can help calm symptoms of asthma. This herb might be useful for those in high-stress fields, such as trading and investment banking.

Milk thistle, an antioxidant, is an anti-aging supplement. Its anti-aging properties stem from its immune system enhancement and anti-inflammatory action. This product can extend life and contribute to a healthier old age. Quantum Brain Healing uses this herb to treat addiction withdrawal, eating disorders, anxiety, and depression. Drug addiction and alcoholism are very damaging to the liver. Eating disorders can result from impaired liver function, where the liver is overactive. A well-functioning liver improves the outcome for many brain diseases. A healthy liver may result in less brain plaque, or amyloid protein deposits in the brain. This may delay or prevent Alzheimer's disease or dementia in some people.

Melatonin for Smoking Cessation

Quantum Brain Healing uses melatonin to help treat depression, along with amino acids, vitamins, minerals, and herbs. Melatonin is a hormone produced in the brain by the pineal gland, from the amino acid tryptophan. It regulates diverse body functions. Melatonin is stimulated by darkness and suppressed by light and is affected by the circadian rhythm. Low melatonin levels are a problem for shift workers. Low levels of melatonin also are associated with breast cancer. Levels of melatonin in the blood are highest prior to bedtime. Melatonin is available as a nutritional supplement. You can also increase melatonin levels by supplementing the amino acid tryptophan.

Melatonin will cross the blood-brain barrier and increase brain circulation. It increases the production of neurotransmitters and balances the brain. It strengthens and enhances the immune system due to the improvement in hormone and neurotransmitter regulation.

Melatonin will help treat depression that stems from inadequate sleep. When the sleep cycle is improved, patients with this type of depression often recover quickly. Anxiety is also a problem when there is sleep deprivation. Almost every type of brain condition gets worse when there is insufficient sleep. It is important to mention the insomnia to your doctor. Hormone imbalances often cause many brain conditions during menopause or andropause (male menopause).

Quantum Brain Healing uses melatonin to treat smoking cessation, insomnia, jet lag, sleep disturbances related to depression, depression caused by sleep deprivation, seasonal affective disorder (SAD), and anxiety. This hormone may be combined with amino acids to increase its effectiveness. Nutritional support can include food-based multivitamins, vitamin E, vitamin D, CoQ10, and alpha lipoic acid. Try adding yoga or mild exercise for producing maximum results from melatonin.

Homeopathy for Drug Addiction

Homeopathy for drug addiction can be useful for those whose addiction is based on deficiency. There are huge fluctuations in the brain's neurotransmitter levels during heroin withdrawal and recovery. An alternative medicine doctor or osteopath may want to test neurotransmitter levels before using Amino Acid Therapy.

The following neurotransmitter may be tested:

> Epinephrine

> Norepinephrine

- ➢ Dopamine
- ➢ Serotonin
- ➢ GABA
- ➢ DHEA
- ➢ Glutamate
- ➢ Histamine

It may take a week or two to receive test results. Acupuncture is a good way to manage fluctuating neurotransmitter levels during this waiting period. Heroin withdrawal causes many problems in several neurotransmitters, including serotonin and dopamine levels. Amino Acid Therapy will administer amino acids to rebalance the dopamine and serotonin neurotransmitters during drug withdrawal; long-term amino acid therapy is recommended. GABA, theanine, glutamine, 5-HTP, and DL-phenylalanine are able to impact your brain's dopamine and serotonin levels.

Heroin acts in the brain like an endorphin to cause pleasure or sleepiness. People get addicted to the relaxed feeling that opiates produce. Amino acids can produce this same relaxed sensation in the body. Therapy uses doses larger than the naturally occurring levels of amino acids found in foods.

Neurotransmitters like serotonin and acetylcholine in the brain may use inositol as a precursor or a cofactor in making more neurotransmitters. Inositol deficiency may produce depression and anxiety. Taking the vitamin inositol may directly enhance neurotransmitters like serotonin.

Useful Homeopathic Remedies for Heroin Addiction

- ➢ Pelargonium reformed is a liver tonic and digestive tonic. Supports good liver function and may help with anger management issues.

- ➢ Nat. sulphuricum (D6) is for people who are even-tempered and sensible but may swing to either end of the spectrum when ill. This reaction may be similar to the extremes experienced during withdrawal and would be good to try during that time.

- ➢ Tarentula (6C) is used for symptoms of hyperactivity, anger, impatience, manipulative behavior, moodiness or wide mood swings, or being antsy. Noise causes person to get worse.

> Kali. phosphoricum helps symptoms of introversion and quietness. This is helpful, as acute fatigue can accompany drug withdrawal.

> Hypothalamus niger treats symptoms of restlessness, or nonsensical, grandiose, paranoid, or hysterical behavior. Reactions are extreme.

> Ferrum phosphoricum helps protective the myelin sheath and can help iron metabolism. Can prevent dizziness, headaches, and restlessness. May help people feel less irritable or tired.

> Magnesium phosphate (Mag. shop. D6) heals frayed nerves; it's an antispasmodic, and nerve and muscle relaxant; it may help relieve stress headaches.

King Homeopathy, based in Asheville, North Carolina, is a great source of homeopathic remedies. It has traditional remedies as well as its own patented products for unusual diseases and underlying weaknesses. Its product line includes miasm homeopathic remedies. These should be tested and treated in people with any type of addiction. Miasms are underlying genetic weaknesses. The ability to recover from most addictions or illnesses will improve after miasms are treated. They can also be treated with retro-viral medications and Nambudripad's Allergy Elimination Techniques (NAET).

Trace Mineral Salt Lithium Orotate

Lithium orotate is a trace mineral salt found in RNA and DNA. It can be used to treat neurodegenerative diseases and repair damaged nerves. Lithium orotate is not a pharmaceutical drug that is marketed by pharmaceutical companies. Trace mineral deficiencies may be contributing factors in many brain illnesses. Trace mineral deficiency may be a result of a disease or a causative factor for a disease or symptom. It is available through your naturopathic doctor or medical physician specializing in alternative medicine.

Lithium orotate mineral salt can treat migraine headaches, but the most unusual use by Quantum Brain Healing for this trace mineral salt is for treating alcoholism and kleptomania. These diseases may benefit from lithium orotate's ability to stabilize neurons, grown new neurons, and increase neural plasticity. Kleptomania is a very difficult disease to treat, and although lithium orotate may not be a cure, it could significantly improve the problems and allow the patient to progress to the point where other treatments could become an option. Any medical treatment that repairs DNA might be helpful in treating kleptomania. Lithium orotate allows the alcoholic patient to reduce their desire for alcohol and may also help ease withdrawal. All trace minerals should be replenished after chelation therapy.

1. Lithium orotate is one of several trace mineral salts that is commonly used in naturopathic medicine. This can travel inside the brain to stabilize many of the chemical activities of the neurons, and it protects brain cells in the hippocampus, striatum, and frontal cortex of the brain. It helps stimulate the growth of new neurons and has the ability to stabilize the brain during periods of extremely irregular brain-wave activity. Lithium orotate can be instrumental in increasing neural plasticity, which is important in preserving or increasing intelligence.

Intravenous Nutritional Therapy, or the Myers Cocktail

The Myers Cocktail is an intravenous therapy that consists of mixing vitamins, minerals, amino acids, and other nutrients. It can be very useful in improving the health of a patient immediately after withdrawal. Most drug addicts are severely deficient in many vitamins and minerals. When nutrients are given intravenously, the digestive system is bypassed, and a much higher level of nutrition can be delivered directly to the cells via the bloodstream. Dr. John Myers was the first doctor to develop an intravenous nutrient therapy that obtained positive clinical results for a variety of medical conditions. This is alternative medicine at its best.

A great example of this type of medicine is Dr. Rick Sponaugle's Florida Detox Clinic located in Palm Harbor, Florida (near Tampa). His clinic is a wonderful resource for Vitamin IV therapy, wellness, and detox from almost any type of drug. It is wellness based medicine and has a great track record in getting patients off drugs and improving their health. He treats patients of all ages. You can make an appointment at 888-775-2770 or online at www.FloridaDetox.com.

The Myers Cocktail improves almost all digestive symptoms, including bloating, diarrhea, food allergies, irritable bowel syndrome, colitis, ulcers, IBS, and Crohn's disease.

The Myers Cocktail intravenous therapy is administered by physicians or nurse practitioners. It improves the body's ability to make energy, and it increases cellular function. You may feel a warm sensation while the IV is administered. The effect is usually fast-acting, but extremely ill people will require several treatments to experience the full effect. I love this therapy.

Emotional Freedom Technique (EFT)

33

Emotional Freedom Technique, or EFT, is a therapy that excels at treating pain or symptoms related to emotional thoughts, feelings, trauma, or addiction. Anxiety, depression, and insomnia related to drug withdrawal can be improved with EFT. This is a fairly inexpensive therapy that can be done with the help of a professional and reinforced by oneself at home. This therapy should be initially performed by an acupuncturist, chiropractor, Orthomolecular Medicine doctor, osteopath, or alternative medicine doctor.

EFT is a relatively new therapy that has not been extensively studied or published, and there are not adequate double-blind studies on this therapy in America. It could benefit many people with disease and emotional trauma, however, as it could alter the electromagnetic field of the patient.

EFT uses fingers to perform a tapping motion on acupuncture points along energy meridians established in Traditional Chinese Medicine. This is called EFT tapping. This process is easy to perform on your own at home, after a medical professional shows you the correct way to do the therapy. The points that are tapped must be exactly correct in location. There may be additional points added to your treatment, depending upon your specific injury, disease, or level of emotional distress. This technique usually must be done more than once in order for it to succeed. Positive and negative affirmations are stated out loud while the tapping is done. It's best to refer to acupuncture charts at home to double-check the correct point locations and to make sure that you are tapping on the desired point.

This therapy can alter thoughts and feelings. Many diseases can improve or be cured when the person changes his or her belief or thought concerning an illness or symptom. Many times, a patient's improvement can be as simple as getting someone to believe he can improve and helping him visualize this change in his life. Tapping may have this ability, along with moving the blocked energy along Chinese energy meridians. These energy meridians correspond to specific organs in the body.

When the body's energy gets blocked or stuck in a specific organ, like the heart or small intestine, it may impact several organs and energy throughout the entire body. Chinese medicine believes that each energy meridian and organ is connected to emotions, directly or indirectly. As energetic blockages are removed and the energy flows freely, the person will improve the symptom, and any emotionally caused problems can heal. It is possible for a person to get well in a single treatment, although many people will require several sessions. EFT will not replace other hard work in overcoming addictions, but it will help in treating addictions and eating disorders. It also can be used for healing depression, stress, anxiety, sleep disorders, migraines, seizures, and tics.

Ondamed

Ondamed is a device that could be considered a combination of neurofeedback for the emotions and an electromagnetic stimulus that energizes electron flow and oscillates cells in a range of .1 to 32,000 Hz. Its intended purpose is to help manage emotional trauma and reduce inflammation and stress. It enhances lymphatic flow, improves metabolism, and affects the nervous system. Frequently, emotional trauma is at the root of addiction. Ondamed may treat hidden emotions that are stored on a cellular level and that negatively affect the immune system.

This treatment may require several sessions for noticeable improvement. You should expect to commit to at least twelve treatments for any addiction. People with more than one addiction may require a longer session and more treatments than those with a single addiction. Tobacco addiction may not be helped with this treatment. Recreational-drug addictions that have been persistent for longer than a decade will require acupuncture with high doses of alpha lipoic acid in addition to this therapy.

Bio-Mat

The Bio-Mat is a device that uses far infrared and amethyst crystals. The patient lies on the mat for twenty or thirty minutes and listens through earphones to sounds and instructions. It seems like a meditation session, and it relaxes your body as the infrared speeds the elimination of toxins. It also ionizes your body with negative ions, which improves your body's ability to heal. The Bio-Mat normally should be used about once a week after the withdrawal period for two months. The Bio-Mat, however, is not inexpensive—it can cost upwards of $2,500, depending on the size you choose, and there is only one manufacturer—but it is a unique device.

ALZHEIMER'S DISEASE

Quantum Brain Healing has many therapies for Alzheimer's disease. These must be administered by a medical or health care professional for the safety of the patient. Major diseases like Alzheimer's may require that the symptoms be handled individually. The strategies for Alzheimer's are to delay onset of the disease, minimize memory loss, increase motor function, improve concentration, calm the patient, improve the energy level, prevent secondary illness, reduce stress, and aid sleep.

Dietary changes should occur and should include an initial detoxification of all heavy metals and pesticides. Serious toxin overload from heavy metals and pesticides may induce Alzheimer's or Alzheimer's-like symptoms. Detoxification can be done with oral chelators and a pure diet. Vitamins, minerals, and orthomolecular amino acid therapy can enhance mental function, improve memory, and increase motor coordination for many patients. Bio-identical hormone replacement therapy can be used to improve energy, concentration, and memory.

Alzheimer's patients should avoid stress, stay hydrated, eat regular meals, and have an organized routine. Remember that these patients are easily upset and very fearful at times. Keep them busy with mental activities, like learning a second language or playing bridge. Dominos, chess, or puzzles also will improve brain function.

Traditional Chinese Medicine herbal formulas, single herbs, and botanical extracts are used to calm the brain and help the memory. Electro-acupuncture, ear acupuncture (with needles or magnets), laser auricular therapy, scalp acupuncture, music therapy, interactive metronome, meditation, yoga, and cranial-electro stimulation with the Alpha-Stim100 are wonderful ways to improve the health and quality of life in this type of patient. Other options include Hyperbaric oxygen chamber, light therapy, Hemi-Sync therapy from the Monroe Institute of Virginia, pulsed energy therapy, electromagnetic medicine, EFT, Transcranial Magnetic Stimulation (TMS), and craniosacral therapy.

Vitamins

Quantum Brain Healing uses vitamin B12 is as a way to improve the brain in several ways. Symptoms of vitamin B12 deficiency include fatigue, brain fog, delusion, poor memory, neurological problems, poor concentration, depression, psychosis, irritability, mania, forgetfulness, and increased sleep requirements. These symptoms may also be indicative of other vitamin or mineral deficiencies. Any of these conditions may be treated with this vitamin if a deficiency of B12 exists. Vitamin B12 is involved in DNA synthesis, and fatty acid synthesis, and it helps break down carbohydrates and covert them into energy. Vitamin B12 directly affects learning skills and memory. Vitamin B12 is found in beef, caviar, chicken, cheese, eggs, fish, lamb, liver, milk, octopus, and shellfish. A sublingual form of this vitamin is available. A multivitamin product should also be taken with this supplement so that the other B vitamins are not deficient.

Orthomolecular Medicine uses higher amounts of vitamin B12 than would be found in multivitamin products or a normal diet. Many brain diseases may require these higher levels of vitamin B12 in order for healing to occur. Alzheimer's disease has several symptoms that can improve with B12, including dementia, depression, long-term memory loss, and impaired ability to convert short-term memory into long-term memory. The other B vitamins should also be included in a vitamin regimen. For nerve injuries and diseases, alpha lipoic acid and high-quality fish oil or cod liver supplements are needed, as is choline or lecithin. Diets for nerve injuries and diseases must include high levels of unsaturated fatty acids.

Nutritional Supplements

Quantum Brain Healing utilizes lithium orotate for treating many diseases, including Alzheimer's disease. Lithium orotate is a trace mineral salt found in RNA and DNA. It can be used to treat neurodegenerative diseases and repair damaged nerves and is commonly used in naturopathic medicine. This trace mineral can travel inside the brain to stabilize many of the chemical activities of the neurons and helps stimulate the growth of new neurons. It protects brain cells in the hippocampus, striatum, and frontal cortex of the brain. It can be useful in many areas of brain stimulation that have been deemed untreatable.

Lithium orotate also can be used for treating migraine headaches and stress-induced memory loss and may help those Alzheimer's patients who have progressed to the point of violent outbursts. It also can be used to treat epilepsy patients and ALS. The medical effect of lithium orotate in both these diseases is similar and may stem from its ability to stabilize the brain during periods of extremely irregular brain-wave activity.

Lithium orotate can be instrumental in increasing neural plasticity, which is important in preserving or increasing intelligence. It may have a use in treating children that are developmentally challenged, but would need to be combined with other treatment options available in Quantum Brain Healing in order to add ten to twenty points to the IQ and rewire the brain. The child would need to be able to verbally communicate in order to try this treatment.

Quantum Brain Healing also uses this trace mineral salt for treating alcoholism. If the Alzheimer's patient is addicted to alcohol, lithium orotate may benefit both issues and allow a long-term alcohol problem to be solved. Additional herbal support should be added for alcohol withdrawal, if this is a problem.

Herbs

Quantum Brain Healing uses botanical extracts, herbal formulas, and single herbs in high doses to treat and heal Alzheimer's disease. Supplements and herbs may be combined with other therapies. There may a focus on removing toxins before beginning the supplements. It is very important to purchase herbs that are free of heavy metals and residue or toxins. Several of the herbs used to treat Alzheimer's are adaptogens and can heal beyond the brain. Adaptogens are substances that can balance the body by stimulating or sedating the underlying medical condition. This is an overly simplified concept of an extremely complex medical concept. These herbs focus on the immune system for improved overall health. It is quite important to have a professional examine the specific herbs you are taking to determine their suitability to be taken together.

Chinese club moss is a very strong and powerful herb that is used for many of the most serious brain illnesses. It is as useful as a pharmaceutical drug for some brain diseases. It can increase energy levels, strengthen the immune system, increase alertness, improve learning, increase memory, impact neurotransmitter levels, and improve nerve function by strengthening and lengthening the nerve impulse. It also can act as a brain enhancer.

Chinese club moss has been used to treat many diseases and conditions, including Alzheimer's disease, myasthenia gravis, Parkinson's disease, memory loss, dementia, and cognitive impairment. Chinese club moss may be useful in reducing symptoms of Huntington's disease, multiple sclerosis, and spastic symptoms of undiagnosed diseases.

Chinese club moss must be combined with a proper diet and large quantities of vitamins and minerals. With Alzheimer's disease, the recommended daily allowance (RDA) of these supplements is insufficient to improve the disease. Very large doses of many vitamins are needed for medicine or herbal products to achieve the best outcome. It is likely that once the body has a major disease, the level of vitamins and minerals needed for basic metabolism is increased. A major detoxification should be implemented early as well. Research is very inconclusive, but many theories conclude that toxic pesticides and chemicals are at the root of diseases and conditions like Alzheimer's, cognitive impairment, early dementia, and unexplained memory loss.

Wild blueberry extract is able to cross the blood-brain barrier and target several areas of the brain, including the cerebellum, hippocampus, and cortex areas. The active ingredients in wild blueberry extract are anthocyanins (antioxidant flavonoids). Wild blueberry extract increases the brain's ability to make more new brain cells and can improve memory and increase learning ability. It also slows the brain's rate of aging and can reverse some signs of aging in the brain and allows brain cells to stay alive longer. Wild blueberry extract is an anti-aging supplement that most people can tolerate easily.

Wild blueberry extract caused brains to have higher levels of dopamine, a brain neurotransmitter that is responsible for controlling body movements and results in better motor control. This extract is an antioxidant and anti-inflammatory for people with amyloid protein buildup in the brain. These people may suffer from dementia or Alzheimer's and wild blueberry extract allows the brain to function more like a normal brain. Adding green tea to the diet of these patients is a great idea to increase brain levels of theanine, improve brain circulation, and increase energy levels. Remember, too, that amyloid protein build up is far less common in people who exercise.

Wild blueberry extract targets oxidative stress and inflammation to reverse aging of the brain that is accelerated by conditions of oxidative stress and inflammation. Bilberry extract is another product that is an antioxidant and anti-inflammatory. Bilberry can increase the life of your brain's cells. A combination of wild blueberry extract with bilberry extract and green tea can improve an Alzheimer's patient's ability to perform motor tasks. These types of supplements need to be incorporated early into the diet of the Alzheimer's disease or dementia patient. These products improve the ability of the brain to covert short-term memory into long-term memory. Wild blueberry extract is an anti-aging and wellness product that has far higher levels of two active antioxidants that locally grown blueberry crops. Wild blueberry extract will allow the aging person to have a better memory, learning ability, and better motor skills.

Gotu kola may be useful in treating Alzheimer's disease. In Traditional Chinese Medicine, this herb is called *ji xue cao*. Gotu kola's ability to enhance brain circulation while reducing inflammation is a major way it treats brain diseases. This herb may interact with blood-thinning agents and should not be taken by those on blood thinners without an Orthomolecular Medicine doctor's care and supervision. Gotu kola is very strong and has properties similar to those found in pharmaceutical drugs. *Do not* take gotu kola without supervision.

Gotu kola has many important actions to help the brain repair itself, including increasing brain circulation and acting as an anti-inflammatory. It is a mild diuretic, so if there is very slight swelling of the brain, it may have a beneficial effect. Brain swelling may occur when there is protein buildup in the brain due to Alzheimer's. Swelling may also occur because of bad circulation in part of the brain. Any swelling in the brain impairs circulation and prevents clear thinking. Gotu kola is also an anti-inflammatory substance that can reduce or prevent inflammation throughout the body. This herb is an adaptogen and can help balance the body. It can stimulate or sedate, depending on the action needed by the body for optimal health. All adaptogens affect the immune system and help the body fight other diseases.

This very effective herb directly affects the cortex of the brain. Gotu kola changes neurotransmitter levels in the brain. Quantum Brain Healing relies on amino acids often to treat GABA levels in the brain for curing and treating depression and eating disorders. Gotu kola can target the GABA receptor sites in the brain and balance neurotransmitter levels. It is essential to remember that any supplement taken to affect neurotransmitter levels must be supervised by a doctor. Do not ever take this type of supplement without informing your health care professional.

Alzheimer's disease can be improved by using the herb hawthorn, a small berry that has been used for centuries. Many other diseases and conditions also are improved with hawthorn, including ADHD, stress, memory loss, arteriosclerosis, ischemia, and stroke. Hawthorn also is commonly used to treat heart conditions, and several serious brain diseases. This herb can be taken as a tea or as a capsule supplement. If there is heart disease, a food-based vitamin and CoQ10 supplement should be added on a daily basis. The Quantum Brain Therapy uses hawthorn and several amino acids to impact the brain's circulation, oxygenation levels, and any inflammation.

Hawthorn can cross the blood-brain barrier and affect the brain directly in many ways, such as increasing blood circulation, lowering blood pressure, and decreasing cholesterol, as well as acting as an anti-inflammatory, antioxidant, and antibiotic to decrease bacteria. Hawthorn's ability to reduce cholesterol is connected to its impact on arteriosclerosis. Insufficient blood flow caused by heart conditions lowers the oxygenation levels in the brain and the impaired blood flow may result in poor brain function and worsens brain illnesses or causes brain illness.

A person with brain and heart disease should include mild exercise or a walking plan as an overall strategy to prevent further problems. This person should also take steps to exclude saturated fats from the diet and include unsaturated fats. Salmon is a great food to include in this person's diet.

Brain diseases might begin when there are heart problems, as the damaged heart's failure to properly oxygenate the brain can cause many problems. A heart condition leads to poor circulation, which may increase the amyloid protein buildup in the brain. The other possibility is that impaired circulation increases stress, and this causes the other brain diseases to manifest. If the Alzheimer's patient had heart problems prior to developing the disease, insist that the doctor test the patient's statin levels. Drugs affecting statin levels may cause the side effect of low CoQ10 levels. Add large amounts Ubiquinol CoQ10 (approximately 300 mg per day) to the other supplements taken by this patient.

Lemon balm, an acetylcholinesterase inhibitor, can help Alzheimer's and Parkinson's patients in the earliest phases of these diseases. It may delay the onset of the disease or prevent mild to moderate dementia. Lemon balm also inhibits the production of the thyroid hormone and could help treat Hashimoto's disease (an autoimmune disease that causes problems with the thyroid) in its early phase. It can also be used to treat hyperthyroid or Graves' disease. Do not take lemon balm if you have hypothyroid disease or take thyroid medicine. Lemon balm acts on the hippocampus area of the brain and functions as an antispasmodic. It is a sedative and antioxidant and can be used to treat stress and anxiety. Its sedative effect can benefit nervous exhaustion. Aging of the brain may be accelerated by bacterial and viral infections, and lemon balm may prevent this.

The herb muira puama should be used in combination with a food-based multivitamin, such as those made by the whole food supplement company Standard Process, to treat Alzheimer's. Muira puama, an antioxidant, is a highly active herb with many active chemical components. This herb crosses blood-brain barrier and increases circulation in several areas, including the hippocampus, cerebral cortex, hypothalamus, and cerebellum areas of the brain and central nervous system. Any herb that acts upon the nervous system can positively benefit almost any condition that affects nerves, including ALS and MS. For Alzheimer's patients, the herb may have use in treating impaired nerve function due to accident or trauma, such as falls.

Muira puama is an adaptogen and can stimulate or sedate, depending on what the person's body requires. It can boost the immune system and is an analgesic that reduces nerve pain because of its analgesic mechanism that can affect the central nervous system. Muira puama is a neuroprotectant; it extends the life of brain cells and enhances memory. Muira puama can treat conditions of stress, depression, and anxiety found in Alzheimer's disease.

Catuaba is a South American herb that has many medicinal properties, including the ability to act as an antibiotic and antiviral. It also is an adaptogen that can sedate or stimulate the brain and central nervous system as needed. Adaptogens often can turn around a difficult disease, such as Alzheimer's, when pharmaceutical drugs have not worked. Catuaba is antioxidant and may be an amino anti-aging herb for the brain. Catuaba is an analgesic for the brain and can calm the brain when overstimulated.

Catuaba should not be considered a sole treatment; rather, it should be combined with nutritional supplements, including amino acids, as a secondary herb. Additionally, 5-HTP, GABA, or SAM-e may contribute to faster balancing of neurotransmitters. Although catuaba is not similar to valerian, it can treat similar diseases and conditions. A liver detoxification prior to the use of catuaba may improve or hasten its success. Quantum Brain Healing relies on the use of therapeutic minerals and vitamins to balance the body. Irregular sleep cycles frequently accelerate the decline of most diseases. The key factor of catuaba is that it is an adaptogen. It sedates the brain and calms the overactive brain to help anger issues present in Alzheimer's disease.

Quantum Brain Healing uses astragalus to enhance immune system resistance and to increase physical endurance. This herb improves mental function in one simple way: a stronger body will support a higher-functioning brain. Astragalus is a wonderful, affordable, anti-aging herb that almost everyone can use at some point in his or her life. Use this herb to reduce stress on an occasional basis to prevent illness. Astragalus fights several types of cancer, including small-cell lung cancer, leukemia, and gastrointestinal cancer. It slows tumor growth and prevents the growth of additional tumors. It can increase T-cell activity.

If you use this herb for anti-aging purposes, you also should take food-based multivitamins; change your diet to organic foods, when available; and include a yoga or exercise program to help balance neurotransmitters and hormones. A well-planned detoxification program, followed up with bio-identical hormones, is also needed. Very few herbs are able to treat eating disorders such as anorexia, but astragalus is the best single herb for this purpose.

Astragalus has antibiotic properties. It is an anti-inflammatory and an antiviral and encourages the body systems to function correctly. It has diuretic properties and increases blood circulation. Many types of blood diseases can benefit from astragalus. It also increases sperm motility and lowers blood glucose. It lowers blood pressure and enhances cardiac function in many ways. Astragalus protects the liver and kidneys, and it may be through this action that astragalus helps prevent senility.

For Alzheimer's patients, astragalus can improve brain issues connected with chronic-fatigue like brain fog, and it can improve learning and increase memory. It can treat dementia and impaired cognitive function. Physical debilitation and brain injury similar to that found in car accidents can be improved in many cases when this herb is taken for about two months. Astragalus may help impaired pituitary function if the pituitary gland is impaired due to inflammation or viral attack, this herb could reverse the condition. It may help patients with diabetes insipidus and could increase the pituitary gland's ability to increase vasopressin levels. *Do not* take this herb without informing your health care professional.

Vinpocetine is a botanical extract that is derived from the periwinkle plant and is very common in naturopathy. This herbal extract has many properties that make it very important in healing the brain. It crosses the blood-brain barrier and acts as a neuroprotectant to protect the brain cells and keep them alive longer.

Vinpocetine is an antioxidant that improves brain circulation and metabolism. It can be used to protect the brain for patients who are subject to strokes and ischemia. After a patient has had a stroke, this extract can be useful in protecting brain cells in the event of a future attack. The extract acts as an anticonvulsant and antismolytic. The anticonvulsant action allows it to reduce seizures in some and prevent seizures in others. This delays the decline for many

Alzheimer's patients. It can prevent atherosclerosis when taken on a long-term basis. It slows or prevents abnormal platelet clumping. Vinpocetine is considered an anti-aging brain supplement. It is not to be used by those taking blood thinners, however, and vinpocetine should not be taken with large quantities of green tea, due to the blood-thinning properties of both vinpocetine and green tea.

Vinpocetine can be useful for many people in treating ischemia, dementia, Alzheimer's disease, Parkinson's disease, seizures, and memory loss. It can also be used as a memory enhancer for those in serious study situations, such as older people returning to college. Vinpocetine may be useful in treating epilepsy caused by traumatic injury. This treatment would be best when tried within one to six months after the injury.

Laser Auricular Acupuncture

Laser auricular acupuncture is successful for some patients with Alzheimer's. The treatments may last approximately twenty-nine to forty-nine minutes. The ear points used to improve Alzheimer's include the brain stem, shen men, brain, occiput, liver, endocrine, cortex, subcortex, heart, spleen, stomach, and large intestine points. The treatments can also be combined with key body acupuncture points like Spleen 4, Spleen 9, and UB 20.

Auricular acupuncture may be less traumatic for younger patients than using body points. The treatments may last approximately twenty-nine to forty-nine minutes. Ten to twenty treatments are needed to achieve results that are sustainable.

Hormone Dysfunction

There is a correlation between hormone imbalance and prognosis for the Alzheimer's patient. Imbalances of estrogen, pregnenolone, progesterone, and testosterone impact the management of this illness.

It is important to get baseline hormone tests results initially. If there is an imbalance in progesterone levels, men and women can correct this by taking the herb vitex. This can also be accomplished with bio-identical hormones of progesterone and testosterone.

Sublingual liquid progesterone may help menopausal women or men over forty with movement disorders impaired by hormone imbalances. Hormone testing must be used before using any hormones. Continuous monitoring of hormone levels is required when taking bio-identical hormones. Be diligent in monitoring the anger levels of the patient - if anger levels are extremely high, this may indicate a high testosterone level. Another way to impact hormone levels is with liquid IV amino acid therapy in your doctor's office, although not many doctors offer this excellent product. It may be available through a physician trained by the American Academy of Anti-Aging Medicine.

Diet

The number-one concern with all brain diseases is that the patient should avoid genetically modified foods (GMF). Several companies have tried to quietly spread GMF across the world, but the European Union has banned GMF. To avoid GMF, try to purchase organic food or grow your own with heirloom seeds. Locally grown produce might be fine, but it is important to question the growers about their seed selection. Farmers' markets also might be an affordable option. Choose organic milk without hormones or antibiotics. Filtered water is always a good choice. These food concepts apply to every diet used for Alzheimer's patients.

Quantum Brain Healing might treat Alzheimer's disease with restrictive diets to alter brain chemistry. The glutamate-aspartate restricted diet (or GARD), rotation diet, elimination diet, macro-biotic diet, and organic diet can improve conditions associated with Alzheimer's disease. GARD is an elimination diet originally developed to treat epilepsy; it identifies foods and ingredients to avoid: gluten, soy, corn, glutamate, MSG, casein, aspartame, and hydrogenated oils.

Gluten is commonly found in wheat and grains. Casein is a protein found in cow's milk and dairy products. Soy is a legume. Corn and all corn products, like corn syrup and corn starch, must be avoided. Many products have corn syrup as a sweetener, rather than sugar. Monosodium glutamate (MSG) is a very common food ingredient in processed foods and often is found in Chinese food. Aspartame is a chemical a sugar substitute known by the brand name of NutraSweet.

GARD restricts glutamate and aspartate nonessential amino acids that stimulate the brain. Glutamate and aspartate are the parent compounds of MSG and aspartame. Aspartame is a well-known neurotoxin and has been connected with brain cancer in Italy. Glutamate and aspartate may cause seizures and may trigger neurodegenerative diseases in some people. GARD allows the gut to heal and recover, due to the removal of gluten, dairy, soy, and corn. These foods may cause damage to the intestinal villi and result in celiac disease or food intolerance. This diet does not restrict carbohydrate consumption; it allows high-glycemic and high-carbohydrate foods. For best results, this diet should be organic, if possible. Refrain from all refined foods, when possible.

Quantum Brain Healing often relies on food-based nutritional supplements for low toxicity and low-cost healing options. Wild blueberries have more nutrients and can treat and prevent memory loss. Locally grown blueberries are one of the most powerful antioxidants for enhancing memory and preserving brain function, but wild blueberries have higher levels of antioxidants.

Heavy-Metals Poisoning

Exposure to heavy-metals may be encountered in water contaminated by drugs, benzenes, chromium, or pesticides, certain foods, the air, the workplace, reclaimed soil, toxic waste sites, refuse disposal sites, and vaccines. Heavy-metals contamination affects the cell's ability to produce energy, its pH level, and electrical charge. Normal cells are alkaline, and cancer cells are acidic. Most viruses cannot live in an alkaline state. Cancer cells become dormant at a pH of 7.4, and they die off when the pH reaches 8.5. Some researchers believe that cancer develops from exposure to heavy metals and International College of Acupuncture and Electro-Therapeutics (ICAET) research by Dr. Yoshimoto Omura shows that there are heavy metals in the nucleus of the many cancer cells. Some cancers may go into remission or be cured with detoxification and immune system stimulation.

We encounter heavy metals—such as aluminum, mercury, lead, arsenic, copper, thallium, and titanium—on a constant basis, and they cause varying symptoms and diseases. Conditions and diseases related to heavy-metals poisoning may include impaired cognitive skills, insomnia, depression, anxiety, stress, ADHD, obsessive-compulsive disorder (OCD), impaired digestion, neuropathy, colitis, delirium, hallucination, fatigue or chronic fatigue, impaired concentration, brain fog, numbness, hair loss, impaired liver function, cancer, weakness, learning disabilities, dementia, and stupor.

Mercury poisoning can cause social withdrawal or interaction problems, depression, mood disorders, aggressive behavior, OCD, autism, insomnia, delirium, hallucinations, chronic fatigue, eating disorders, suicidal threats, ADHD, weakness, fatigue, colitis, speech problems, difficulty walking, temper tantrums, hearing loss, convulsions, seizures, birth defects, spontaneous abortion, motor problems, rashes, skin problems, nausea, vomiting, diarrhea, stomach cramps, allergies, asthma, and neurological problems.

Aluminum poisoning can cause Alzheimer's, fatigue or chronic fatigue, weakness, dementia, skin problems, rashes, motor disturbances, neurological problems, allergies, asthma, infertility issues, and respiratory diseases.

Lead poisoning can cause memory problems, concentration difficulty, depression, mood swings, irritability, insomnia, sleep disturbance, anxiety, eating disorders, ADHD, mental retardation, impaired intelligence, birth defects, spontaneous abortion, neurological problems, convulsions, seizures, headaches, muscle pain, hypertension, cardiac problems, and suppressed immune function.

The skin is a major organ through which the body detoxifies. Our body also filters toxins from the blood system (detoxification) through the liver, kidneys, gallbladder, and the lymphatic system. It is important to detoxify these systems by drinking plenty of pure water. There are several ways to reduce the heavy-metals load on the body, including diet, nutritional supplements, intravenous chelation therapy, far infrared sauna, foot ionizing detoxification, hot yoga, and any exercise that produces sweat.

IV chelation therapy can be administered in a doctor's office, usually over several hours. It involves injecting ethylenediaminetetraacetic acid (EDTA) into the bloodstream to remove heavy metals, chemical toxins, mineral deposits, and fatty plaques. EDTA is a synthetic amino acid chelating agent for most metals other than mercury. DMSA and DMPS are chemicals used intravenously to chelate mercury but are not approved by the FDA.

Oral chelator nutritional supplements can be found in vitamin shops. The nutritional supplements that function as oral chelators include cilantro, organic barley, organic wheat grass, organic alfalfa, kelp, seaweed, chorella, alpha lipoic acid, L-cysteine, methionine, vitamin C, garlic, methylsulfonylmethane (MSM), and pectin. Citrus fruits are good choices because they are high in roughage and can push heavy metals out of the large intestine and speed elimination. It is very important to drink large quantities of water when using oral chelators of any type, including food therapies.

NeuroCare

This medical device is a therapeutic electric stimulator and should never be confused with neurofeedback devices or brain-stimulating devices. The system uses high voltage to treat many brain illnesses, including depression, insomnia, anxiety, and addictions. Its' other medical uses include diabetic wound care, muscle atrophy, paralysis from trauma, post-surgical recovery, prevention of deep vein thrombosis, and increasing local circulation. The treatment of Alzheimer's disease will require eight to twelve months' treatment, but it is possible to notice improvement after a single session. Cost of the NeuroCare device exceeds the price of many competing medical device products, but treats several brain diseases.

Music Therapy

Quantum Brain Healing relies on a large group of supplements, including amino acids, vitamins, minerals, and herbs. This is integrated into an overall program that includes detoxification of chemicals, toxins, and pesticides for many patients. After the toxins are removed, a healthy diet of organic vegetables and fruits will help people regain health quickly. Food-based multivitamins are included for most people.

For some people, this is not enough and adjunct therapies will be used in mass for very hard cases. Metatones is auditory vibrational energy therapy that addresses problems for learning disabilities, autism, addiction, depression, insomnia, ischemia, and Alzheimer's disease. The brain can be balanced with amino acids to assist with neurotransmitter rebalancing, and auditory therapy can also indirectly affect neurotransmitter levels.

Music therapy, Acutonics (sound healing education), singing, and Tibetan singing bowls are simpler versions of the concept of using music or sound vibrations to heal. The Hemi-Sync method is a more sophisticated version of vibrational sound therapy developed by Dr. Robert Monroe. The Monroe Institute is now run by Skip Atwater. The brain can be balanced by auditory therapy. The sounds are played on a CD and listened to with headphones. The brain-wave activity is altered by the sound vibration as it is heard. There are several types of brain waves, and your brain may not experience proper brain-wave activity. The Hemi-Sync method adjusts your brain-wave activity.

Research shows that Parkinson's and Alzheimer's patients' brains have decidedly different brain waves than the normal brain. Hemi-Sync works to entrain the brain into the proper brain-wave activity for health. Vibrational energy healing is based on the tenet that disease stems from a lack of proper resonance. This is relatively inexpensive treatment—just the cost of the CDs—and you can play the CD's as many times as you need. Although it might seem unusual therapy and sound therapy have many successful results. Most forms of medicine believe that disease is rooted in a lack of balance.

Health will return when cells are put into vibrational balance. It seems that music therapy may be one more way in which to influence and change neurotransmitter levels. Classical music and baroque music are the best type for balancing the brain. Music therapy with a harp has been used to treat MS. Singing upbeat songs is a great way for an Alzheimer's patient to improve his or her depression and participate in a group activity. Stroke patients who are unable to speak may be able to hum along with music.

Reflexology

Reflexology is based on the principle that the anatomy of the body is reflected in miniature reflex zones on the head, ears, hands, and feet. Reflexology treatment, which involves pressure, is most commonly applied on the foot to heal the body. Reflexology promotes relaxation and reduces stress. Both feet are worked on, one at a time, during the course of a full session.

The reflexologist will gently massage your feet and apply pressure to the reflex points that correlate to your health problems. With Parkinson's disease, pressure is applied to the points on the foot that correlate to the head, brain, brain stem, pituitary, pineal/hypothalamus, heart, liver, and thyroid. Reflexology s similar to the concept of acupressure. Some reflexologists apply pressure with their fingers, while others use small instruments.

People with foot problems, such as like severe calluses or corns, should visit a podiatrist for treatment prior to a reflexology treatment. Sessions typically last sixty minutes. Because Parkinson's is a chronic disease, it would require many treatments. Many reflexologists believe that manipulation of the feet reduces the lactic acid accumulation in the tissues and releases tiny calcium crystals that accumulate in the nerve endings of the feet. Another way to reinforce this action on the feet is to purchase an infrared foot massager. Foot ionizing detoxification also may help remove calcium and lactic acid buildup from your feet.

Reflexology restores the qi, or free flow of energy, from the feet to the corresponding organs. Some reflexologists believe that pressure on the reflex points may trigger the release of hormones, including endorphins, which are chemicals in the brain that naturally block pain. Reflexology creates relaxation, improves circulation, and increases the rate at which detoxification occurs. Reflexology can help control seizures for some patients, but there are no major clinical research trials to verify the effectiveness of reflexology. Reflexology should be used in addition to other therapies.

Bio-Mat

The Bio-Mat is a device that uses far infrared and amethyst crystals. The patient lies on the mat for twenty or thirty minutes and listens through earphones to sounds and instructions. It seems like a meditation session, it relaxes your body, and the infrared speeds the elimination of toxins. It also ionizes your body with negative ions, which improves your body's ability to heal. The Bio-Mat normally should be used about twice a week on the Alzheimer's patient. The Bio-Mat, however, is not inexpensive—it can cost upwards of $2,500, depending on the size you choose, and there is only one manufacturer—but it is a unique device.

rTMS

Repetitive transcranial magnetic stimulation (rTMS) is a noninvasive method for applying electromagnetic fields to the brain. Application is through a medical device with a low 0.9 hertz frequency stimulation. It requires more than one session to be effective. One of the side effects of rTMS is a tendency to underestimate time. Another side effect may be a slight headache. Use of rTMS is contraindicated in epilepsy and multiple sclerosis.

It would be very helpful if Alzheimer's patients were given detoxification for heavy metals and pesticides prior to administering the rTMS. Oral chelation, with formulas available in health food stores, and products like rutin, chorella, organic wheatgrass, organic barley capsules, aloe, parsley, garlic, and alpha lipoic acid will safely remove toxins over time. It will take approximately six to twelve months to remove most of the toxins found in a middle-aged adult. Saunas can accomplish this with about three to twelve sessions lasting about thirty minutes. The rTMS may be used approximately one month after aggressive oral chelation has started.

Single sessions of rTMS placed over the temporal or temporoparietal cortex can cure a very short-term problem with tinnitus (ringing in your ears). Repeated sessions of rTMS may successfully treat tinnitus, but the treatment is not known to cure tinnitus. The results are variable. It may have more success for those whose problem is due to long-term effects of drug addiction. This treatment may also be used in some forms of hearing loss that are not noise-induced. Hearing loss from medications and diseases may find some help with rTMS.

This treatment affects the auditory cortex and may help other problems associated with the auditory cortex, including auditory hallucinations, Parkinson's disease, memory problems in the motor cortex, flashbacks, and depression. When it was tested in patients with major depression, using the therapy five times per week, it was successful. It is very difficult to treat major depression successfully, and this may not be one of the best options. This treatment is noninvasive and causes no pain. It may have results that extend beyond the motor cortex area of the brain.

Some studies indicate that this treatment increases brain plasticity and could have the ability to increase intelligence, given the optimal combination of brain nutrients and other alternative therapies. This treatment also may be a way to enhance learning and increase memory, and it could be wonderful for those who have memory and learning disabilities connected to Parkinson's disease, head trauma, brain injuries, ischemia, or memory loss due to cardiac problems from low oxygen levels in the brain. These are areas of medicine that very difficult to manage and treat.

ANXIETY

Nutritional supplements, amino acid therapy, yoga, vitamins, herbal patent medicine, single herbs, acupuncture, electromagnetic therapy, EFT, and bio-electric stimulation therapy (BEST) are therapies that can help depression and anxiety. Quantum Brain Healing strives to find the most cost-effective and fastest treatment for each patient. This is based on medical diagnostic tests, patient history, and physical examination.

Whenever your doctor gives you an examination, key visual signs indicate vitamin deficiencies. These include cracks around your lips, dark circles under your eyes, ridges or spots on your fingernails, dry skin, and other changes that must be noted in your medical chart. Do not leave your doctor out of your nutritional supplement and alternative therapy selection process. Get his perspective, but make your own decision and always keep him in the loop, with your treatment choices noted clearly in your medical records.

Anxiety can have significant consequences—it can impair relationships and careers. Prior to the invention of modern antidepressant and anxiety medications, opioids were used to treat anxiety and depression. Now anxiety can be treated successfully with alternative medicine.

Anxiety disorders may result from hormone and neurotransmitter imbalances—there may be chemical reactions in the body that prevent neurotransmitters from working with the receptor sites in the brain, which may be due to an underproduction of the brain's natural painkillers. Severe anxiety can be helped with treatment for this underproduction.

Using the opioid-blocking drug naloxone for several days to one week can interrupt the body's irregular brain cycle. Research shows that when these neurotransmitters are prevented from acting with naloxone, people fail to become accustomed to initially frightening stimuli. Their reaction increases rather than decreases. Brain scans showed this activity in the amygdala, the brain area that processes fear. The amygdala affects the limbic structure, including the basal ganglia, which serve to alert the body and set the level of anxiety.

Hyperactive basal ganglia function is found in anxiety disorders. Valium for three to five days might achieve a similar result as naloxone, but for a different reason. The key to alternative medicine is to focus on supplements and medical devices that target the limbic area.

Anxiety may benefit from many types of stimulation. Several factors influence the doctor's anxiety therapy of choice, such as the length of time the patient has suffered from anxiety, the patient's age, and the dietary habits and use of natural supplements.

Visualization can also be utilized to alter the firing rate in the limbic area of the brain and can significantly lower anxiety. Studies show that many people who use visualization can change the rate of neuronal firing in the brain. They imagine stimulating a brain part, and this may positively alter the brain activity for most people, although this could impact the brain negatively if done incorrectly. There are several visualization methods for altering the firing rate and changing the dominant brain activity from the amygdala to the prefrontal cortex. Neurofeedback software also could be useful to achieve this goal.

Three amino acids are used in Quantum Brain Healing to heal and treat anxiety. Large doses of these can repair the imbalance in the brain and reproduce many brain chemical effects that are similar to those achieved with medicine or drugs. Try to treat anxiety and stress by avoiding these during your daily routine. Do not rely on medications long term for treating anxiety. Many therapies and medical devices can help and will allow you to forego dependence on medications.

Avoiding long-term use of medications is especially important because many people who suffer from anxiety also suffer from addictions. People with anxiety disorders, post-traumatic stress disorder (PTSD), physical abuse, or sexual abuse suffer higher-than-average opiate addiction rates. They frequently turn to heroin. People who have experienced high levels of fear and threat often are attracted to drugs that allow them to relive the effect of exaggerated emotions.

It is imperative to biochemically balance the brain while calming the emotions when treating anxiety disorder. It is also helpful to treat anxiety disorder at its earliest symptom. Anxiety, stress, and depression are often accompanied by eating disorders, especially binge eating. This is likely the patient's attempt to manipulate the brain biochemically through food. All food produces chemical reactions in the body that impact the brain. The person with anxiety is attempting to alter his or her body chemistry but is failing to achieve the changes that would balance the brain. Additional brain destabilization often occurs during this period. Those who suffer from anxiety should focus on improving their diet and avoiding unneeded over-the-counter drugs.

Anxiety may often be caused by negative interpersonal relationships with bosses, friends, children, parents, coworkers, employees, maids, yardmen, or spouses. It's often helpful to try to relate to these people in another way. If the problem occurs over breakfast or during a Monday morning staff meeting, for example, reschedule interactions for later in the day. Each person has a particular biorhythm, and some times of the day are better for interaction. It's also a good idea to limit discussion of stressful topics to a set amount of time, such as ten minutes.

People who regularly engage in exercise or meditation experience less anxiety. Their bodies age more slowly, and they experience less disease. Those who schedule yoga, tai chi, qi gong, ballet, golf, biking, hiking, or walking on a regular basis at least four days per week—will achieve a healthy body and mind.

Insomnia—several nights without adequate sleep—can contribute to anxiety in most people, yet anxiety also causes insomnia. If you suffer from insomnia, you may need to invest in a new mattress, especially if yours is more than twelve years old. New hypoallergenic pillows and sheets made from organic fabrics may be beneficial for some people. A ceiling fan may help a room with inadequate air flow. It also might be good to try an air ionizer from Sharper Image, which removes particles and dander from the air. It is also important for the air filter in the air conditioning system to be cleaned or replaced. You can also try to remove any old or moldy carpets. Clean any mold or fungus on the wall or air conditioning register with bleach.

You also might want to spray hydrogen peroxide in the kitchen and bathroom air-conditioning vents. You can't be too careful about keeping mold and fungus under control in areas of the house that have water in the room.

Amino Acid Therapy

Amino acids, herbs, or precursors to neurotransmitters can be used to target similar outcomes as antidepressants. 5-HTP is initially converted into serotonin and later into melatonin. Phenylalanine is converted into tyrosine. Tyrosine and SAM-e are initially converted into dopamine. Dopamine can be converted into norepinephrine or epinephrine. GABA, L-theanine, and L-tryptophan can also be converted into neurotransmitters and affect moods.

Dietary L-lysine deficiency increases stress-induced anxiety. In one small study, L-lysine supplementation lessened plasma cortisol in response to stress and reduced chronic anxiety. L-lysine acts like a partial serotonin receptor antagonist, inhibiting neurotransmitter re-uptake in the synapse. The bottom line is that L-lysine can reduce stress and chronic anxiety in people who have deficiencies of the amino acid.

Orthomolecular Medicine uses theanine, SAM-e, and 5-HTP to help the body lower anxiety. L-lysine can be used for chronic anxiety. Your doctor will recognize the difference between chronic anxiety and casual anxiety. If you have been in a situation such as an earthquake or fire, you may have chronic anxiety. These amino acids should be taken on a daily basis for several months and may be needed for several years for the body to balance. Periods of extreme stress may increase the amount needed. Certain life events increase anxiety, including major promotions, additional responsibility (such as a board of directors position), remarriage, children, a new house, retirement, a death in the family, major illness, and layoffs. These events may require the addition of another amino acid or herb to handle this increased anxiety.

Insomnia and sleep disorders may improve with melatonin. A calcium, magnesium, and vitamin D combined supplement is another sleep inducer for some patients. The amino acids 5-HTP and theanine may help other people sleep better. Theanine is a great amino acid treatment for those suffering from anxiety. 5-HTP is a great amino acid treatment for some types of depression, while GABA is better for other patients suffering from depression. Purified fish oil is great for many people suffering from depression, skin problems, and sleep disorders. Organic coffee may help some people with extremely mild depression. Many years ago caffeine was a treatment for mild depression. Another very inexpensive way to treat depression is to drink bergamot tea. This is the most cost-effective product available in America and the UK.

Anxiety can often be improved in about one week to three weeks by taking 5-HTP at doses of 50–300 mg three times a day. The dosage is dependent on the patient's weight, size, age, and physical condition. The 5-HTP increases the body's serotonin level, and it may be taken with food. Any insomnia associated with the depression may improve significantly. 5-HTP may not work for everyone and may cause slight nausea. Do not use 5-HTP in combination with drugs that increase serotonin (SRRIs).

SAM-e is another amino acid that will work alone for many people to resolve depression within two to three weeks. Take 400 mg of SAM-e before bed on an empty stomach as an effective way to resolve depression. SAM-e should be taken for four to six weeks before deciding on its effectiveness.

Many supplements—including melatonin and a combination of calcium, magnesium, and Vitamin D—can alleviate anxiety. For supplements to be effective, however, they must be the best quality nutritional products. Other methods for combating anxiety include eating yogurt, cottage cheese, milk, or dairy products to get calcium in your daily diet. Warm milk can be sipped at night before bed to help you sleep. Having sex helps people fall asleep. Avoid large quantities of alcohol when there is a sleep disorder, as alcohol impairs the brain-wave activity during the night.

Anxiety, depression, and sleep disorders may be related. Simple anxiety may resolve itself when sleep patterns have normalized. Depression often will improve when the patient is able to sleep eight hours per night.

Do not assume that insomnia or anxiety is the disease; these can be symptoms of disease. Cardiac issues cause sleep problems for some people. Chinese herbal formulas are an excellent way to treat cardiac issues with natural medicine. This type of sleeping problem can be improved with the herbal product of hawthorn berries or the amino acids arginine and orthinine. CoQ10 will further stabilize and support cardiac function. If you have undiagnosed cardiac issues and cannot sleep well, you may need to have your heart evaluated. Poor oxygen content in your blood or a partially functioning mitral valve may cause you to wake up in the middle of the night. Alcoholism also is a huge cause of insomnia and should be dealt with quickly.

Herbs

Quantum Brain Healing uses many herbs to treat anxiety including St. John's wort, passionflower, valerian, kava kava, lemon balm, Bacopa monnieri, hops, skullcap, ashwagandha, and ginkgo biloba. Below are examples of how these herbs have a capacity to treat the brain.

Kava kava will sedate the overactive brain and heal anxiety, but it is important not to overuse this herb. Kava acts on the limbic system, and it affects several neurotransmitters, including GABA and noradrenaline. The limbic area of the brain is key to your emotions of sadness, fear, and anger. Kava is an anxiolytic and may be used to treat anxiety. It can enhance cognitive thinking skills and improve reaction time. Kava is effective for treating anxiety, nervousness, stress, and insomnia—these conditions are related for many people, and kava's slight sedating effect may resolve anxiety and stress. Kava also successfully treats agoraphobia; this may be tied to its ability to affect the limbic area of the brain. It is an anti-inflammatory and can be considered a secondary level anti-aging herb. It can act as a muscle relaxant on the skeletal muscles and central nervous system.

Kava may be an adaptogen due to its slight ability to elevate mood and sedate. Frequently, herbs that produce two opposing actions, depending on what is needed by the body, are considered adaptogens. According to a study at the University of Aberdeen in Scotland, kava is associated with lower levels of leukemia and ovarian cancer. It is important to note, however, that there are reports of severe liver toxicity by a few who have used this herb. This may be due to problems with how the kava is made or other substances that the patients are consuming while on this herb. Kava is not recommended for those with Parkinson's, liver disease, lung disease, depression, or bipolar disorder. Kava has negative interactions with acetazolamide, amiloride, or furosemide, or with angiotensin-converting enzyme (ACE) inhibitors, such as benazepril, captopril, lisinopril, quinapril, ramipril, levodopa-based medication, alcohol, Xanax, barbiturates, or other mood-altering drugs. It is contraindicated in these cases.

Kava must be supported with vitamins, minerals, and high levels of antioxidants. A break should be taken from this herb on a regular basis. Consume a variety of organic vegetables and fruits, and avoid alcohol, cigarettes, nicotine, and recreational drugs when taking kava. Do not do anything to overload the liver with drug toxins, cleaning chemical residues, food dyes, food additives, or artificial sweetener toxins. A regular liver detoxification is a good idea for anyone taking kava.

Lemon balm is a sedative and antioxidant that can be used to treat stress and anxiety. Its sedative effect can benefit nervous exhaustion. This herb also acts on the brain in many ways to reduce signs of aging. Aging is accelerated by high levels of stress, poor sleep, poor diet, increased occurrence of disease. Aging of the brain is accelerated by bacterial or viral infections that go undiagnosed and untreated. Any herb that has antibiotic and antiviral actions may be taken on an occasional basis to prevent brain aging. Green tea also falls into this category.

Quantum Brain Healing utilizes the skullcap herb for many brain diseases that require calming or sedating a part of the brain. Skullcap and Orthomolecular Medicine may be useful in speeding the balancing of neurotransmitter levels. Most brain diseases are rooted in the basis of unbalanced neurotransmitters. Amino acids can quickly rebalance the neurotransmitter levels when the correct ones are chosen and the correct ratio of amino acids is used. This is difficult to achieve for those medical professionals without experience in Orthomolecular Medicine. Scutellaria lateriflora, or the skullcap leaf, has sedative, anticonvulsive, and anti-inflammatory effects on the brain. This herb has been used in America for hundreds of years. This is not a Chinese herb.

Skullcap herb may be used to treat brain disease, including epilepsy, ADD, headaches, neuralgia, insomnia, hysteria, anxiety, delirium, and convulsions. Skullcap can be used in addiction disorders for symptoms like withdrawal from barbiturates, alcohol, and tranquilizers. This Quantum Brain herb should be used in an overall treatment plan for those suffering from addictions. Preventing brain disease and protecting the brain is an important step in your anti-aging program. It is possible to take at least twelve to twenty biological years from your brain. This will allow you to work longer and perform complex tasks with ease.

The European herb piracetam acts on the brain in many ways. These medical actions include increasing brain circulation, increasing cholinergic receptors in the brain, enhancing memory, and acting as a neuroprotectant. This actually alters the functioning of the right temporal lobe. Piracetam may be used in treating many brain diseases, including amnesia, anxiety, dyslexia, senility, and Alzheimer's. Anxiety often increases when any brain disease occurs. Many patients with diseases that affect the right temporal lobe of the brain can take piracetam and monitor its impact for an improvement in their right temporal lobe. The brain diseases need many other therapies in addition to piracetam for the optimal treatment.

Nutritional Supplements

Quantum Brain Healing uses melatonin to help treat depression, along with amino acids, vitamins, minerals, and herbs. Melatonin is a hormone produced in the brain by the pineal gland from the amino acid tryptophan. It is available as a nutritional supplement. You can also increase melatonin levels by supplementing the amino acid tryptophan. Melatonin is stimulated by darkness and suppressed by light, and it is affected by the circadian rhythm. It regulates diverse body functions. Levels of melatonin in the blood are highest prior to bedtime. Low levels of melatonin are associated with some types of cancer.

Melatonin will help treat depression that stems from inadequate sleep. Anxiety levels frequently increase with too little sleep. When the sleep cycle is improved, this type of anxiety or depression patient will often recover quickly. Adequate sleep allows the body time to repair DNA damage during the night and produce new cells. This is how the body repairs itself from illness and injury. Sleep allows you to regain your health from most diseases and illnesses.

Anxiety can stem from waking up in the middle of the night from hormone and neurotransmitter imbalances. Tachycardia can cause you to wake up at night. Alcohol levels can impact sleep and waking up in the middle of the night. Blood sugar swings can cause you to wake up . Almost every type of brain condition gets worse when there is insufficient sleep. It is important to ask your doctor how to resolve this problem. Hormone imbalances often cause many brain conditions during menopause or andropause.

Melatonin will cross the blood-brain barrier and increase brain circulation. It increases the production of neurotransmitters and balances the brain. It strengthens the immune system. The enhanced immune system is due to the improvement in hormone and neurotransmitter regulation.

Quantum Brain Healing uses melatonin to treat anxiety; it's also used to treat insomnia, jet lag, ischemia, smoking cessation, sleep disturbances related to depression, depression caused by sleep deprivation, and seasonal affective disorder (SAD). This hormone may be combined with amino acids to increase its effectiveness. Nutritional support can include food-based multivitamins, vitamin E, vitamin D, CoQ10, and alpha lipoic acid. Yoga or mild exercise will help produce maximum results from melatonin.

The treatment of anxiety, as well as depression and sleep disorders, must focus on removing or reducing tobacco products, alcohol, caffeine, and cocaine. Dark chocolate that is 70 percent chocolate can have a noticeable stimulating effect on some people. Do not eat chocolate or drink tea immediately before bed due to the caffeine content. Practicing yoga can improve anxiety, depression, and sleep disorders. Yoga's effects often can be seen within one month. Walking several times per week also can help resolve anxiety and depression.

Heavy-Metals Poisoning

Heavy-metals poisoning creates many health problems. Toxin exposure may be encountered in bad water, food, air, the workplace, reclaimed soil, toxic waste site, refuse disposal sites, and vaccines. Conditions and diseases related to heavy-metals poisoning may include impaired cognitive skills, insomnia, depression, anxiety, stress, ADHD, obsessive-compulsive disorder (OCD), impaired digestion, neuropathy, colitis, delirium, hallucination, fatigue and chronic fatigue, impaired concentration, brain fog, numbness, hair loss, impaired liver function, cancer, weakness, learning disabilities, dementia, and stupor.

Mercury poisoning can cause social withdrawal or interaction problems, depression, mood disorders, aggressive behavior, OCD, autism, insomnia, delirium, hallucinations, fatigue and chronic fatigue, eating disorders, suicidal threats, ADHD, weakness, speech problems, colitis, difficulty walking, temper tantrums, hearing loss, convulsions, seizures, birth defects, spontaneous abortion, motor problems, rashes, skin problems, nausea, vomiting, diarrhea, stomach cramps, allergies, asthma, and neurological problems.

Aluminum poisoning can cause Alzheimer's disease, fatigue and chronic fatigue, weakness, dementia, skin problems, rashes, motor disturbances, neurological problems, allergies, asthma, infertility issues, and respiratory diseases.

Lead poisoning can cause memory problems, concentration difficulty, depression, mood swings, irritability, insomnia, sleep disturbance, anxiety, eating disorders, ADHD, mental retardation, impaired intelligence, birth defects, spontaneous abortion, neurological problems, convulsions, seizures, headaches, muscle pain, hypertension, cardiac problems, and suppressed immune function.

The skin is a major organ through which the body detoxifies. Our body also filters toxins from the blood system (detoxification) through the liver, kidneys, gallbladder, and the lymphatic system. It is important to detoxify these systems by drinking plenty of pure water. There are several ways to reduce the heavy-metals load on the body, including diet, nutritional supplements, intravenous chelation therapy, far infrared sauna, foot ionizing detoxification, hot yoga, and any exercise that produces sweat.

IV chelation therapy is administered in a doctor's office, usually over several hours. It involves injecting ethylenediaminetetraacetic acid (EDTA) into the bloodstream to remove heavy metals, chemical toxins, mineral deposits, and fatty plaques. EDTA is a synthetic amino acid chelating agent for most metals other than mercury. DMSA and DMPS are chemicals used intravenously to chelate mercury, but are not approved by the FDA. The nutritional supplements include cilantro, barley, wheatgrass, alfalfa, kelp, alpha lipoic acid, L-cysteine, methionine, vitamin C, garlic, MSM, and pectin.

Many doctors will request that patients include a mild form of exercise, such as yoga, gardening, walking, biking, or volleyball to manage and prevent anxiety. This is especially true for children who suffer from depression. Children with depression should be encouraged to be socially active. Older patients can walk or do mild exercise in their chair. Chi machines will improve circulation for patients who may not be able to walk. Patients lie on the floor and put their legs onto a machine, which moves their legs in a slow motion from side to side. Swimming can be another option, but it is important to watch for chlorine allergies. It is also important to pay extra attention to the diets of children and older patients. Any dietary allergies or environmental allergies can create stress and anxiety.

Treatment choices for depression may include the following:

➤ Alpha-Stim 100, an electrical stimulation device that clips onto the ear lobes

➤ acupuncture electro-stim attaches electrical stimulation to acupuncture needles

➤ electrical stimulation of the auricular acupuncture points with a hand held electrical stimulation device

➤ medical-grade laser therapy on auricular acupuncture points

➤ magnetic stimulation of auricular points with small retention magnets

Laser Acupuncture

Auricular laser therapy is quite useful in treating many types of neurological disorders. Brain stem injuries resulting from trauma, surgeries, falls, accidents, and inflammatory diseases can be improved and treated with auricular laser therapy. Many types of brain diseases can be improved, including Parkinson's and Alzheimer's, by using auricular laser therapy. Cognitive disorders and poor memory can be improved for many people with this therapy. Mild learning disorders caused by autism and ADD also can be improved with this treatment.

This therapy is needed two or three times per week for two or three months with a monthly follow-up treatment. Long-term illnesses often require long-term care. This therapy can reduce or eliminate the need for medicine for some patients. The office visits for this therapy may last from twenty to forty minutes. Your alternative medicine doctor will add nutritional supplements to your diet while you are on this therapy. The worst symptoms of the disease may also require oral detoxification products to remove toxins from your liver.

Milk thistle is a great herb for most people and helps reduce toxins in the liver. Most patients take this herb for seven to twelve weeks. Spanish black radish supplements produced by Enzymatic Therapy are very good for improving liver health. Organic alfalfa, alpha lipoic acid, pectin, organic wheatgrass, and garlic supplements also are very good detoxification agents. Fasting with juice or pure water can reduce toxins for the young and healthy. Fasting is not recommended, however, for those with serious brain diseases. Hot yoga or Bikram yoga will reduce toxins. You must drink large quantities of pure water during any detoxification. You can remove years of damage to your liver with a carefully monitored detoxification.

The auricular acupuncture points used in the laser treatment on your ear include the brain, cortex, subcortex, liver, sympathetic, zero point, shen men, spleen, large intestine, small intestine, yang or pituitary, heart, stomach, and triple burner points. Laser auricular therapy will not hurt. It is needle-free; the skin is penetrated by the laser beam traveling under the surface of the skin. If you are nervous, please advise your doctor. He or she can add an additional acupuncture point, named yin tang, to reduce your anxiety.

Emotional Freedom Technique (EFT)

Emotional Freedom Technique, or EFT, is a therapy that excels at treating pain or symptoms related to emotional thoughts, feelings, trauma, or post-traumatic stress disorder (PTSD). Anxiety and depression can be improved with EFT. This is a fairly inexpensive therapy that can be done with the help of a professional and reinforced by oneself at home. This therapy should be performed initially by an acupuncturist, chiropractor, Orthomolecular Medicine doctor, osteopath, or alternative medicine doctor.

EFT is a relatively new therapy that can benefit many people with disease and emotional trauma. It could alter the electro-magnetic field of the patient. This therapy has not been extensively studied or published; however, there are not adequate double blind studies on this therapy in America.

EFT uses fingers to perform a tapping motion on acupuncture points along energy meridians established in Traditional Chinese Medicine. This is known as EFT tapping. This process is easy to perform on your own at home after a medical professional shows you the correct way to do the therapy. The points that are tapped must be exactly correct in location. There may be additional points added to your treatment, depending upon your specific injury, disease, or level of emotional distress. This technique usually must be done more than once in order for it to succeed. There are positive and negative affirmations that are stated out loud while the tapping is done.

This therapy can alter your thoughts and feelings. Many diseases can improve and heal when the person changes his or her belief or thought concerning an illness or symptom. Many times, a patient's getting better can be as simple as getting someone to believe he can improve and helping him visualize this change in his life. Tapping may have this ability, along with moving the blocked energy along Chinese energy meridians. There are several energy meridians in the body, and they correspond to specific organs.

When the body's energy gets blocked or stuck in a specific organ, like the heart or small intestine, it may impact several organs and energy throughout the entire body. Chinese medicine believes that each energy meridian and organ is connected to emotions directly or indirectly. As energetic blockages are removed and the energy flows freely, the person will improve, and any emotionally caused problems can heal. It is possible for a person to get well in a single treatment, but many people will require several sessions. EFT will not replace hard work in overcoming addictions. It will help in treating addictions and eating disorders. It can be used for healing depression, stress, anxiety, sleep disorders, migraines, seizures, and tics.

EMDR

Eye movement desensitization and reprocessing (EMDR) helps treat emotional issues and all types of anxiety caused by automobile accidents, assault, natural disasters, sexual assault, personal failures, such as demotions at the office or divorce. It may help someone who is not helped by the typical psychologist or psychiatrist.

EMDR is performed by a professional, and it usually more than one time to relieve severe anxiety. The doctor must initially analyze the patient's current situations that trigger an emotional disturbance and evaluate past traumatic events. He must determine if the patient currently has the needed coping skills to prevent any similar circumstances from arising. If the patient has the skills, then the doctor may move forward.

A specific memory or event is identified and processed using EMDR procedures. The patient identifies the most specific image related to the memory and any negative feelings of self-worth that are tied to this event. This is processed along with the patient's sensations and feelings that are tied to this event. These feelings may include fear, nausea, headaches, crying, trauma, and inadequacy. The patient is given a positive image and belief to substitute for the problematic feeling or event. The intensity of the negative emotions should diminish during this treatment and a positive emotion will root the patient.

The doctor helps the patient focus on the event and negative feeling while body sensations are created. The patient moves his eyes rapidly and follows the doctor's fingers as they move for approximately thirty to sixty seconds. All doctors use the eye movements, and some doctors may add auditory sounds and tapping similar to Emotional Freedom Technique (EFT). The doctor asks the patient to describe the sensations that are being processed. This therapy can work wonders for people who experience massive amounts of fear and physical trauma.

Reflexology

Reflexology promotes relaxation and reduces anxiety and stress. A reflexologist will work on both feet, one at a time, during the full session. The reflexologist gently massages your feet and applies pressure to the small areas that correlate to your health problems. These correlate to all the organs, glands, and body parts. Pressure is applied to the organs affected by the disease and to the associated area of the disease. The reflexologist should massage the areas associated with the head, brain, brain stem, adrenals, liver, spleen, gallbladder, stomach, heart, and adrenal glands.

Reflexology performed by an acupuncturist will include the use of the acupuncture points on the feet for a more complex and complete treatment. The reflexologist will treat one foot first, then the other. Some reflexologists apply pressure with their fingers, while others use small instruments. Sessions typically last from thirty to sixty minutes. Acute anxiety may require five treatments, and chronic anxiety will require twelve to nineteen treatments. The nerve endings for the body are in the feet. Massage can calm the nervous system and relieve stress and anxiety. Many reflexologists believe that manipulation of the feet reduces the lactic acid accumulation in the tissues and releases tiny calcium crystals that accumulate in the nerve endings of the feet. This restores the qi, or free flow of energy, from the feet to the corresponding organs. Many believe that pressure on the reflex points may trigger the release of hormones, including endorphins, chemicals in the brain that naturally block pain. Reflexology creates relaxation, which improves circulation. Reflexology speeds the body's rate of detoxification. This treatment can help anxiety and insomnia.

Aromatherapy

Aromatherapy is the controlled use of essential oil in treating anxiety, stress, and many brain disorders. It may be utilized by itself or as an adjunct therapy to other mainstream and alternative medical treatments. Traditional Chinese Medicine uses herbal remedies in an oil base that are very similar to essential oils in the treatment of arthritis, muscular strain, and back pain due to circulatory problems. Naturopathy uses essential oils for many illnesses.

Lemon balm, California poppy, chamomile, lavender, rose, and bergamot essential oils can be used to treat anxiety and stress. These essential oils can affect the levels of neurotransmitters or the amount of time they reside in the brain. They also might affect the manner in which a neurotransmitter interacts with its receptor site in the brain disease. Lemon balm may help prevent the loss of the key brain chemical acetylcholine. The lemon balm is incorporated into a base oil, like grape seed oil, and is rubbed on the face, stomach, and feet for a six-week period, after which there may be significant improvement. Lemon balm reduces agitation in patients. Citrus essential oils like bergamot and orange may affect the same and additional neurotransmitter levels.

In the morning, lemon oil can be used in a diffuser to help patients wake up and increase alertness. In the afternoon, chamomile essential oil can be used in a lotion base, or several drops may be added to a washcloth to calm patients and reduce agitation.

Homeopathy

Homeopathy is an alternative form of medicine that was developed in the early 1800s. It was common prior to the development of Western medicine. A number of different homeopathic remedies treat disease; these are differentiated by symptoms. For the best outcome, it's important to find a knowledgeable practitioner. The varying outcomes may be affected by your doctor's talent in providing you with correct remedy, as well as your own immune system. Homeopathy seeks to stimulate the body's defense mechanisms and processes to prevent or treat illness. Some people respond very quickly to homeopathy, and others may never improve with this treatment. Homeopathy uses a diluted substance to treat a person. This dilution, or "remedy," would cause the illness or symptom if it were given at full strength. Homeopathic remedies are relatively inexpensive and may be another tool to use on difficult cases.

Discontinue taking any remedy if there has not been improvement after one week and/or seek another opinion. There are homeopathic products for sale online and at various natural food stores, such as Whole Foods or Central Market. You also can find an extensive line of products online at http://QuantumBrainHealing.com. Some homeopathic practitioners will custom-make remedies for each person. A visit with a medical practitioner who has some training in homeopathy would prevent mistakes.

The following homeopathic remedies may be useful for addressing short-term anxiety and chronic anxiety:

➤ Aranea diadema   neuralgia, insomnia in alcoholics

➤ Avena sativa   mental exhaustion

➤ Coffea cruda   excessive mental activity, insomnia

- Delphinium staphisagria — neuralgia
- Kalium bromatum — nervous system disorders
- Moschus moschiferus — dizziness, neurosis
- Mygale lasiodora — anxious, restless
- Nux moschata — mental illness, hysteria
- Picrinicum acidum — severe mental fatigue, possibly due to grief
- Spigelia anthelmia — migraine, neuralgia
- Stannum metallicum — neuralgia, nervous disorder
- Zincum metallicum — extreme mental exhaustion, brain fatigue, irritable

AUDITORY HALLUCINATIONS

Quantum Brain Healing treats auditory and visual hallucination patients with a varying degree of success. Any type of hallucination is very difficult to treat, and is quite important to locate the trigger for the initial event. If the event is physical, such as poisoning, medication, automobile accidents, or traumatic head injuries, the doctor can treat the root cause. Root causes of poisoning may require radical shifts in diet and chelation therapy. Heavy-metals poisoning can cause many health problems, but these toxins will respond to detoxification strategies.

Several categories of patients experience hallucinations. Patients with schizophrenia, bipolar disorder, post-traumatic stress disorder (PTSD), and depression may experience auditory hallucinations. The University of Manchester, England, researched a connection between childhood abuse and auditory hallucinations in bipolar patients and found there is a significant connection. Seventy percent of auditory hallucinations occur after physical or sexual abuse, an accident, or the death of loved one. The voices in auditory hallucinations seldom respond to medication. PTSD and depression patients should read my suggested treatments for those diseases. My online articles on PTSD and depression treatment offer many suggestions. The underlying diseases associated with hallucinations are very serious and need to be addressed separately from this symptom.

Brain locations involved in auditory hallucination are Wernicke's area, which is a part of the left temporal lobe, which is involved in perceiving, spoken speech, and a similar area of the right temporal lobe. In addition to the temporal lobe differences, altered neural pathways also are associated with auditory hallucinations. These different neural pathways may be minor changes for adults with late onset of hallucinations, rather than for those people with early onset of schizophrenia or bipolar disorder. Minor changes may have some success with pursuit of changing brain plasticity through cognitive enhancement techniques. The use of scalp acupuncture may enable brain plasticity to increase with a long-term treatment plan. It takes a long-term treatment of acupuncture for hallucinations to resolve themselves.

Researchers haven't found the specific neural mechanisms at work with hallucinations. Brain scans indicate the areas of the brain that process sound and store memories activate at a higher level during auditory hallucinations. This may indicate that the excitatory neurotransmitters are out of balance and the inhibitory neurotransmitters need to be stimulated or supported in some biochemical fashion. Amino acid therapy could be utilized for this purpose. Yoga and meditation alter neurotransmitter levels in a slow manner. Many diseases are associated with auditory hallucinations: sleep deprivation, schizophrenia, bipolar disorder, post-traumatic stress disorder, depression, alcohol withdrawal, cocaine abuse, stimulant abuse, delirium, dementia, temporal lobe epilepsy, familial temporal lobe # 4 epilepsy, Gelineau's syndrome, and familial type 1 hemiplegic migraine.

Hallucinations also can be associated with high doses of cocaine, amphetamine, or other stimulant. Drug abuse causes nutritional problems like undereating and overeating. Drug abuse also directly interferes with sleep. People with bipolar disorder, depression, and schizophrenia often abuse recreational drugs, and the genesis of their auditory hallucinations may be drug-related. Avoiding recreational drug use may improve auditory hallucination. Detoxification of drug residue from the liver and fat stores of the body can bring further improvements.

High caffeine intake is somewhat correlated with auditory hallucinations. Discontinuation of caffeine may reduce the intensity or frequency of auditory hallucinations.

Hallucinations can be treated successfully only when underlying diseases are treated and all substance abuse stops. Always talk to your doctor about drug abuse, alcohol abuse, nicotine abuse, and caffeine abuse if you suffer from hallucinations. One or more of these issues may be the root cause of the disease. The toxin buildup in the body from these substances can have a serious impact on many diseases over the long term.

Quantum Brain Healing offers many solutions for hallucinations, including Orthomolecular Medicine with herbs, vitamins, amino acids, and minerals. It is important to look at the complete medical situation of the patient before treatment. Underlying diseases must be diagnosed and treated along with the hallucination. The patient needs brain-functional MRI tests, along with kidney and liver tests. Brain neurotransmitter testing is a good choice. Hormones may need to be tested but are unlikely to be the root cause. Extreme hormone imbalances may contribute to hallucination, but it would be wise to look for tumors in the brain and auditory area. Tumors along the optic nerve or in the brain could be associated with visual hallucination. Poisoning also may be connected with visual hallucination. Severe oxygen deprivation to the brain can result in hallucinations.

Chinese patent herbal formulas, along with scalp acupuncture, can be effective for this condition. Auricular acupuncture can be successful with the use of retention needles. Electro-stimulation in acupuncture should be used with care. Moxa also should be used very carefully. Use a far infrared heating lamp with spray moxa on the bottom of the feet for fifteen to twenty-five minutes if there is serious energy deficiency or the patient is older than age 70. Discontinue any therapy which has a negative impact on symptoms. At least ten treatments of acupuncture should be taken before this therapy can be appropriately evaluated. As mentioned, hallucinations are difficult to treat. Never give up after one treatment of any type of alternative therapy, assuming that it does not work. With many brain diseases, progress will be slow.

Auricular Therapy

Auricular therapy treats the entire body with acupuncture points located on the ear. This alternative medicine therapy mobilizes endorphins and Menkalinan opioid peptides, increases serotonin and dopamine neurotransmitters, and increases levels of substance P and cholecystokinin (CCK). Auricular therapy can stimulate or sedate depending on which ear points are selected and how long the session lasts. Auricular acupuncture helps the body balance its levels of stress and sex hormones. It helps reduce cortisol and glucose levels and allows the body to reduce its overall inflammation level. Auricular therapy modulates neurotransmitters and is very helpful in dealing with substance-abuse recovery and mood disorders. Auricular therapy can be used in addition to acupuncture on the body and scalp.

Auricular therapy can include needles, electrical stimulation, laser therapy, or electro-acupuncture. Opiate withdrawal symptoms can be reduced within fifteen minutes of application of auricular therapy to certain auricular acupuncture points by applying electrical stimulation to the ear. It can be used to treat addiction to cocaine, crystal meth, methadone, morphine, alcohol, opiate, food, sex, and nicotine.

The National Acupuncture Detoxification Association (NADA) established five auricular points for treating addiction issues. NADA protocols are offered in over five hundred clinics worldwide, including America, Europe, Australia, and the Caribbean. Yale University has conducted research on the effectiveness of the NADA protocol for cocaine, heroin, and methadone addiction.

The five NADA auricular acupuncture points are included in the addiction points:

> Shen Men: stress, anxiety, excessive sensitivity

> Autonomic Point: balance sympathetic and parasympathetic nervous systems, blood circulation

> Liver: hepatitis, cirrhosis

> Lung 2 addiction lung issues

> Kidney

> Hearing

> Large Intestine

This treatment protocol creates higher levels of optimism and cooperation in patients, improved sleep, fewer cravings, less stress and anxiety, and reduced need for drugs. Patients who successfully completed conventional treatment with the combined with auricular therapy showed the fastest recovery with the highest abstinence rates.

The highest success rates were those patients who received auricular therapy five times per week over a sixty day period. Acupuncture improves patient compliance, mood, and physical symptoms. It is relatively low cost and produces very few side effects.

Ozonated Drinking Water

A water purification system, which may be hardwired under the kitchen sink or used next to the kitchen faucet, could be quite useful. Although it is a fairly expensive item—the kitchen model may cost $1,200 to $2,500—it produces pure water that has been ozonated and is alkalizing in nature. The water may be able to improve conditions in the body associated with high acidity levels. There is little research for this technology—other than that many diseases (including cancer and Alzheimer's) get far worse with high levels of acidity in the body but this type of water may enhance water metabolism through the body and alter energy production rates.

Drugs or heavy-metals toxins often are the underlying cause of auditory hallucinations. Quantum Brain Healing begins with detoxification of toxins and heavy metals, along with orthomolecular amino acid therapy. It incorporates vitamin IV therapy with acupuncture for twenty treatments. Detoxification may resolve many hallucinations for patients with high levels of heavy metals, toxins, and pesticides, and the patient may get completely well after detoxification and acupuncture. Substance abuse *must* be eliminated in order for patients to become and remain healthy.

Heavy-Metals Poisoning

Heavy metals poisoning creates many health problems. Toxin exposure may be encountered in bad water, food, air, the workplace, reclaimed soil, toxic waste site, refuse disposal sites, and vaccines. Conditions and diseases caused by heavy-metals poisoning may include impaired cognitive skills, insomnia, depression, anxiety, stress, ADHD, obsessive-compulsive disorder (OCD), impaired digestion, neuropathy, colitis, delirium, hallucination, fatigue and chronic fatigue, impaired concentration, brain fog, numbness, hair loss, impaired liver function, cancer, weakness, learning disabilities, dementia, and stupor.

Some researchers believe that cancer develops from exposure to heavy metals. Heavy metals such as aluminum, mercury, lead, arsenic, copper, thallium, and titanium are encountered on a constant basis. Research shows that there are heavy metals in the nucleus of the many cancer cells. The heavy-metals contamination affects the cell's ability to produce energy, its pH level, and electrical charge. Normal cells are alkaline, and cancer cells are acidic. Most viruses cannot live in an alkaline state. Cancer cells become dormant at a pH of 7.4, and they die off when the pH reaches 8.5. Some cancers can go into remission or be cured with detoxification and immune system stimulation.

Mercury poisoning can cause social withdrawal or interaction problems, depression, mood disorders, aggressive behavior, OCD, autism, insomnia, delirium, hallucinations, fatigue or chronic fatigue, eating disorders, suicidal threats, ADHD, weakness, speech problems, colitis, difficulty walking, temper tantrums, hearing loss, convulsions, seizures, birth defects, spontaneous abortion, motor problems, rashes, skin problems, nausea, vomiting, diarrhea, stomach cramps, allergies, asthma, and neurological problems.

Aluminum poisoning can cause Alzheimer's, fatigue or chronic fatigue, weakness, dementia, skin problems, rashes, motor disturbances, neurological problems, allergies, asthma, infertility issues, and respiratory diseases.

Lead poisoning can cause memory problems, concentration difficulty, depression, mood swings, irritability, insomnia, sleep disturbance, anxiety, eating disorders, ADHD, mental retardation, impaired intelligence, birth defects, spontaneous abortion, neurological problems, convulsions, seizures, headaches, muscle pain, hypertension, cardiac problems, and suppressed immune function.

The skin is a major organ through which the body detoxifies. Our body also filters toxins from the blood system (detoxification) through the liver, kidneys, gallbladder, and the lymphatic system. It is important to detoxify these systems by drinking plenty of pure water. There are several ways to reduce the heavy-metals load on the body, including diet, nutritional supplements, intravenous chelation therapy, far infrared sauna, foot ionizing detoxification, hot yoga, and any exercise that produces sweat.

IV chelation therapy is administered in a doctor's office, usually over several hours. It involves injecting ethylenediaminetetraacetic acid (EDTA) into the bloodstream to remove heavy metals, chemical toxins, mineral deposits, and fatty plaques. EDTA is a synthetic amino acid chelating agent for most metals other than mercury. DMSA and DMPS are chemicals used intravenously to chelate mercury, but are not approved by the FDA. The nutritional supplements include cilantro, barley, wheatgrass, alfalfa, kelp, alpha lipoic acid, L-cysteine, methionine, vitamin C, garlic, MSM, and pectin.

Diet

Quantum Brain Healing focuses on detoxification early in treatment and uses several types of detoxification, including far infrared sauna, ionizing foot detox, oral chelators, and the brown-rice detoxification diet. The brown-rice diet is a very inexpensive and easy diet for detoxification. Many health problems arise from the average diet in the industrialized world. It is high in refined foods, meat, fat, sugar, caffeine, chemicals, dyes, and alcohol. This results in a very acidic body pH.

It is critical to attain a pH balance near 7.0 to achieve the biochemical state necessary to heal most diseases. Heavy-metals detoxification accelerates as blood chemistry is improved. The brown-rice diet can reduce or eliminate many symptoms, such as arthritis, allergies, sinus problems, obesity, skin problems, headaches, chronic pain, digestive issues, and liver problems. Many brain disorders are made worse with bad diets. This diet is beneficial in determining the significance of your diet's effect on your brain disorder. It is not a cure-all, however, and should be avoided by diabetics. Check with your health care practitioner prior to starting this diet if you have a serious health problem. If your symptoms drastically improve, you may assume that you either are allergic to some food you consume on a frequent basis, or there is a chemical or metal exposure that may require further medical attention.

It is very important to detoxify on an annual basis and lower your body's chemical and heavy-metals load. The best way reduce your toxic load is to include other detox therapies when you do a diet cleanse. These can include hot yoga, foot ionizing detoxification, far infrared sauna, and exercise. Anything that makes you sweat will help remove chemicals and heavy metals. The brown-rice diet is preferable to water fasting or the Master Cleanse for toxin removal for most people. The Master Cleanse is a fasting diet that may bring on some serious side effects for people in poor health or older patients. It is a specific diet that has several books written about it.

The brown-rice diet can be well tolerated for one to two weeks. Eat brown rice cooked in pure spring water for five small meals of brown rice in order to stabilize glucose levels stable. If you like the flavor of the herb cilantro, add it to the cooking water of the rice. This will accelerate heavy-metals removal. Drink a minimum of six to ten glasses of purified mineral or spring water, fresh vegetable juice, and herbal caffeine-free tea each day. It is fine to add barley or wheatgrass in liquid or tablet form to these drinks. This will also increase heavy-metals removal.

Another diet that is good for detoxification is a raw fruit and vegetable diet. Do not use the Master Cleanse for a prolonged period if your goal is heavy-metals detoxification. The toxin overload can occur due to heavy metals being excreted from your body. This can make you feel sick.

Quantum Brain Healing follows detox with dietary changes, including the elimination of caffeine, artificial sweeteners, and food additives, and it introduces an organic diet high in fresh vitamins and minerals. Whole food-based multivitamins and anti-aging supplements, like CoQ10, resveratrol, and alpha lipoic acid can improve overall health quickly. Green tea taken every day is another good anti-aging drink. Dietary changes should include organic decaf coffee, reduced refined foods, spring water, organic fruits, and organic vegetables. Oral chelators can be introduced into the diet on a frequent basis to help prevent the hallucinations from recurring after treatment. Oral chelators include pectin, organic barley tablets, organic wheatgrass tablets, cilantro, milk thistle, pectin, garlic, and chlorella. It is very important to keep the diet clean in order to treat this symptom successfully.

Far infrared sauna should be done twice per week for one month, followed by one treatment every week to two weeks for fourteen weeks. Foot ionizing detox can be substituted for about one-third of the far infrared sauna treatments. Foot ionizing detox can be done without much stress while sitting in a chair. Oral chelators can be taken for a nine-month period. Oral chelators include pectin, cilantro, garlic, chlorella, selenium, vitamin C, vitamin E, milk thistle, malic acid, vitamin B12, organic wheatgrass tablets, organic barley tablets, organic aloe vera juice, alfalfa capsules, Patented Cilantro Product by Dr. Omura, and alpha lipoic acid. The addition of a whole food-based multivitamin should be incorporated into the diet.

Essential fatty acids are frequently insufficient in the diet of a person with auditory hallucinations. The essential fatty acids needed are GLA, borage oil, omega-3, and omega-6. Try to include a variety of essential fatty acids into your diet by eating salmon, almonds, walnuts, Brazil nuts, avocados, pecans, olive oil, hazelnuts, pistachios, sunflower seeds, and pumpkin seeds.

Sleep Issues

Trauma and sleep deprivation of an extended and serious nature may also trigger auditory or visual hallucinations. Quantum Brain Healing uses meditation, yoga, melatonin, 5-HTP, valerian, hops, lemon balm, and St. John's wort to help induce sleep safely. After the sleep cycle is regulated, the auditory hallucination should quickly fade.

Any sleeping area should have a reduced electromagnetic field due to wireless interference from computer systems and telephone systems. It is imperative to remove wireless telephone systems from the patients' homes. Wired telephone systems or fiber optic systems are acceptable.

Herbs and Botanical Extracts

Vinpocetine can be useful for many people in treating auditory hallucinations, brain fog, fatigue, depression, short-term memory loss, long-term memory loss, headaches, vertigo, excessive fear, amnesia, anxiety, and stress. It can also be used as a memory enhancer for those in serious study like graduate school. Its brain-enhancing characteristics include improving concentration, alertness, creativity, memory, and increasing the rate of learning. It may help auditory hallucination patients through its ability to calm the brain.

Vinpocetine is an antioxidant that improves brain circulation and metabolism. After a patient has a stroke, this extract can be useful in protecting brain cells in the event of a future attack. It can reverse speech impairment and mental decline in stroke patients. The extract acts as an anticonvulsant and antismolytic. This anticonvulsant action allows it to reduce seizures in some and prevent seizures in others. It may delay decline for patients and reduce the severity of the hallucinations. It also may slow the frequency of occurrence. It reduces the confusion associated with dementia and Alzheimer's disease. It can reduce cholesterol or plaque in the brain. It can remove or chelate several heavy metals. Vinpocetine is considered an anti-aging brain supplement. It is not to be used, however, by those taking blood thinners, fish oil, green tea, or any blood-thinning substances.

The calming nature of skullcap assists brain issues of over stimulation or interrupted brain signals. Scutellaria lateriflora, or the skullcap leaf, has sedative, anticonvulsive, and anti-inflammatory effects on the brain. Skullcap may be used to treat brain disease, including auditory hallucinations, epilepsy, ADD, headaches, neuralgia, insomnia, hysteria, anxiety, delirium, and convulsions. Skullcap can be used in addiction disorders for withdrawal from barbiturates, alcohol, and tranquilizers.

Nambudripad's Allergy Elimination Techniques (NAET)

Nambudripad's Allergy Elimination Technique (NAET) eliminates allergies of all types and levels, using a blend of medical therapies taken from acupuncture or acupressure, allopathy, chiropractic, nutrition, and kinesiology. It can be non-invasive when acupressure is utilized. It is pain-free, but there may be the presentation of allergic symptoms during the twenty-five hour period following the treatment. For optimal treatment, the patient needs to be rested, hydrated, and not hungry. There is usually an avoidance period of twenty-five hours after the treatment where specific items need to be avoided. These items or foods will be identified for the patient at the time of treatment.

NAET can be used to treat and improve many brain illnesses. Most diseases are impacted by environmental or food allergies. Auditory hallucination patients should be treated for allergens. If NAET is not used, some other form of allergy testing and treatment must be tried to address the triggers for this condition. This will boost the immune system and improve the patient's prognosis, although it will not work on all the people. NAET will require about two or three treatments per week over a period of approximately one year, with each treatment lasting approximately fifteen to forty-five minutes. The severity of the case and the age of the patient will determine the number of sessions required.

NAET treats one allergen is treated at a time. Auditory hallucination will require many treatments before it can be determined if this therapy will help reduce the number of hallucinations. Auditory hallucination patients have immune systems that are under attack, and the immune system is more likely to be overactive than deficient. Any additional symptoms, such as depression, anxiety, insomnia, memory loss, nicotine addiction, and alcoholism will require additional attention and treatment. A person with auditory hallucinations may have many allergies, and it could take about one hundred office visits to clear the substances triggering the immune response. These substances include pesticides, heroin, cocaine, pot, cigarettes, food dyes, artificial sweeteners, alcohol, air pollutants, medicines, antibiotics, home building materials, mold, mildew, and foods. Anyone who has been exposed to Agent Orange or sarin gas should consider NAET as a great opportunity for some men to recover from the many side effects of serious poisons.

Inform your doctor exactly where you have been in the world and which type of toxins may have been present. Do not expect each doctor to ask this question. You must volunteer this information and initiate this conversation.

Basic essential nutrients are treated and cleared during the first few visits. It is important to diagnose and treat the primary allergens that negatively affect the body's ability to maintain health. The longer an allergy goes untreated, the more inflammation occurs. Ordinary items that are not allergens will cause a reaction in a body that is in a state of high inflammation. Extremely ill people with many allergies may require an extended period to get well, but some improvement should be noticeable after the initial twenty-five treatments.

NAET can treat many diseases, including brain illnesses, cancer, autoimmune diseases, and diabetes. Diseases improve when NAET is used to reduce allergenic inflammation throughout the body. Chronic illness usually requires more treatments to produce desired results. Acute situations, such as food poisoning, can respond within two hours. The website to locate a trained NAET practitioner anywhere in the world is http://www.naet.com.

Transcranial Magnetic Stimulation

Transcranial magnetic stimulation (TMS) and repetitive transcranial magnetic stimulation (rTMS) utilize magnetic coils close to the surface of the head to generate magnetic pulses. These pulses pass through the skull and influence activity in the underlying brain region. TMS is used as a research tool and as an experimental therapy for promoting recovery after stroke and for treating depression and migraine.

Research was done at Yale for auditory hallucinations including severe and constant voices that were treated with TMS. This therapy places an electromagnet on the scalp, which generates a moderate magnetic field pulse. The magnetic pulses penetrate the skull and stimulate the cerebral cortex. Low frequency TMS induces sustained reductions in cortical activation. Low-frequency TMS reduces the experience of auditory hallucinations.

Approximately half of the patients experiencing this treatment had excellent results.

TMS is currently under development, and research is being conducted to move this device toward smaller devices, so we can expect changes. Non-steroidal herbs that have similar medical actions might be used in conjunction with TMS, as this may speed the recovery. The brain of a person with auditory hallucinations is overstimulated and may need to be sedated with drugs or herbal formulas. TMS devices have had inconsistent results for some patients, but this may be due to the length or frequency of the treatments. Stimulating the right prefrontal cortex improves symptoms of depression and anxiety, but can also increase aggression, undesirable risk-taking behavior, or anger.

Repetitive transcranial magnetic stimulation (rTMS) is a noninvasive method for applying electromagnetic fields to the brain. Application is through a medical device with a low 0.9 hertz frequency stimulation. This treatment requires more than one session. One of the side effects is a tendency to underestimate time. Another side effect may be a slight headache. It is contraindicated for those who have epilepsy or multiple sclerosis.

Single sessions of rTMS placed over the temporal or temporoparietal cortex can cure a very short-term problem with tinnitus (ringing in your ears). Repeated sessions of rTMS may successfully treat tinnitus, but the treatment is not known to cure it. The results are variable. It may have more success for those whose problem is due to long-term effects of drug addiction. This treatment may also be tried for some forms of hearing loss that are not noise-induced. Hearing loss from medications and diseases may find some help with TMS.

This treatment affects the auditory cortex and may help other problems associated with the auditory cortex, including auditory hallucinations, Parkinson's disease, memory problems in the motor cortex, flashbacks, and depression. It was tried on patients with major depression five times per week, and there was success. This treatment is noninvasive and causes no pain. The treatment may have results that extend beyond the motor cortex area of the brain.

Hemi-Sync

Hemi-Sync involves binaural beating, a sensory-information stimulus, and changes the information sent to the reticular-thalamic activating system that improves attention, focus, and level of awareness. Hemi-Sync signals contribute to a greater balance of activity of the brain's right and left hemispheres and cortical and subcortical areas. Hemi-Sync is used to improve auditory hallucinations, learning disabilities, developmentally disabled, ADHD, OCD, brain trauma, bipolar disorder, and to improve cognitive function. Do not use this therapy if you have a unilateral hearing loss. Hallucinations caused by events in a war may respond well to this therapy. This therapy may need to be tried nine times before you may notice significant improvement. Do not use this therapy more than once if your hallucinations become worse.

Alpha-Stim 100

This small medical device is prescribed by doctors and acupuncturists; it is slightly larger than a deck of cards. It has wires that attach to ear clips. Each ear clip has a small pad where several drops of a liquid are placed before the clips are attached to your earlobes. The time and frequency on the machine are set at your prescribed levels. The device operates with a D battery and may be worn several times per week. Auditory hallucinations require a very low frequency setting and a small amount of time on the device. This should be tried for no more than nineteen minutes during its initial use. If there is pain, lower the frequency setting. If this does not remove the pain, discontinue wearing the device, and inform the doctor immediately. It has not been tested for this use. This device has been tested in small clinical trials in several VA Hospitals for several different medical uses. It is very good at altering neurotransmitter levels and has been tried for controlling seizures.

Aromatherapy can be tried as a method to calm the brain. The essential oil used must have calming aromas, such as rose, lavender, and edelweiss. Relieving hallucinations requires several types of alternative therapy for some patients.

Hallucination alternative therapies include:

➢ Detoxification

➢ Ozonated water purification system for the kitchen

➢ Organic diet

➢ Vitamin IV therapy

➢ Aromatherapy

➢ Orthomolecular therapy with amino acids

➢ Scalp acupuncture

➢ Chinese patent herbal formulas

➢ Herbs

➢ Hemi-Sync by the Monroe Institute

➢ Auricular acupuncture

➢ Scalp acupuncture

➢ Group cognitive therapy

➢ Alpha-Stim 100

AUTISM SPECTRUM DISORDER

There are no clear answers for the origin of autism and Asperger's syndrome. There has been a significant rise in the disease, but this may be due to many reasons. Theories about the origin of autism include bacterial infections, viral infections, genetic weakness, vaccine exposure, environmental toxins, and heavy-metals toxicity.

Many allegations attempt to tie the autism spectrum syndrome to vaccines in young children, as the diagnosis usually occurs when children are young. This may be the case, or the vaccine may trigger the disease in a child with a challenged immune system. A deficient immune system can react to a multitude of triggers, such as chemicals, pollutants, foods, dyes, medications, and environmental allergens. One-third of autistic children suffer from epilepsy. Emotional trauma for a child with a compromised immune system may provide the mechanism for symptoms of autism to occur or worsen.

There may be many dietary issues involved in autism. Immune system deficiencies may enable relatively safe substances to produce large negative events in patients. Several theories have evolved from the basis that much disease is a result of allergies. After the allergies are cleared, the disease or symptoms disappear. NAET incorporates this concept into its method of healing by clearing allergies. The rotation diet, elimination diet, gluten-free diet, and casein-free diet are other examples of how to reduce food allergies.

Every autistic child should have allergy tests and diagnostic testing for vitamin and mineral deficiencies. Autistic children are often deficient in selenium, lithium, and cholesterol. Vitamins and nutritional supplements should commence after the test results are in hand.

Alternative treatments to help autism include:

- Neurofeedback
- CES
- EEG biofeedback
- Auricular therapy
- Scalp acupuncture
- Chinese herbal formula
- NAET

- Music therapy
- Sound therapy
- Tomatis Method or listening therapy
- Interactive metronome therapy
- Herbs
- Epsom salt baths
- Chiropractic
- Repeated transcranial magnetic stimulation (rTMS)
- Orthomolecular Medicine
- Hemi-Sync by the Monroe Institute
- Radionics
- BEST
- Osteopathic manipulation
- Craniosacral therapy
- Auditory integration training (AIT)
- Vibrational medicine
- Dietary changes
- Nutritional supplements
- Elimination diet
- Rotation diet
- Gluten-free diet
- Applied behavioral analysis (ABA)
- Hyperbaric oxygen
- Heavy-metals detoxification
- Play therapy
- Homeopathy
- Stem cell therapy
- Animal play therapy

- ➢ Secretin hormone therapy
- ➢ Treating fungal infections to improve gut health

Nutritional Supplements for Autism:

- ➢ Aloe vera
- ➢ Vitamin B12
- ➢ Vitamin C
- ➢ Selenium
- ➢ Choline
- ➢ Probiotics
- ➢ Intravenous vitamins
- ➢ Digestive enzymes
- ➢ Omega-3 fatty acids
- ➢ Omega-6 fatty acids
- ➢ Calcium
- ➢ Melatonin
- ➢ DHA oil
- ➢ Alpha lipoic acid (low doses)
- ➢ Chorella
- ➢ Organic wheatgrass
- ➢ Lithium orotate (trace mineral salt)

Heavy-Metals Toxins

Scientists Schneider, Leong, and Syed have demonstrated how mercury and heavy metals pass through the blood-brain barrier to infiltrate the brain cells and disturb normal cell growth. Some children are more affected than others. Chelation therapy can provide a mechanism for removal of the heavy metals from the brain and allow it to heal. Nutritional supplements and a good toxin-free diet are necessary after the chelation therapy in order for a complete healing to occur.

Dr. Townsend of the Townsend Letter, the physician author of a monthly alternative medicine newsletter by subscription, has identified that American children are exposed to heavy metals through vaccine exposure. In their first two years of vaccines, children are exposed to 237 micrograms of mercury. The current EPA safe level of mercury for a child is one-tenth of a microgram/kilogram per day. Dr. Townsend has identified the following vaccines as dangerous for young children with weakened immune systems:

> ➢ Hepatitis B contains 12 mcg of mercury; this is thirty times the safe level.

> ➢ DTaP and HiB vaccines given on the same day contain 50 mcg of mercury; this is sixty times the safe level.

> ➢ Hep B, polio vaccines contain 62.5 mcg of mercury, which is seventy-eight times the safe level.

> ➢ At fifteen months, the child receives another 50 mcg of mercury, which is forty-one times the safe level.

Chelation therapy—either intravenous and oral chelation—is a technique that removes heavy metals from the body. The intravenous chelation therapy is expensive and takes several hours for each treatment. It usually requires between twenty and thirty treatments. Oral chelation is slower but gentle and less expensive. I would recommend small amounts of oral chelation for children. It is important to err on the side of caution when the ability of the patient to communicate is limited. Oral chelators used by physicians include DMSA (sodium 2,3 dimercaptorpropane-1-sulfate) and EDTA (ethylenediaminetetraacetic acid).

Contaminated seafood and fish are a common source of heavy metals. There also can be heavy-metals contamination in products produced in other countries with few or unenforced health codes. Foods that can contain sulfur can reduce heavy metals. These include garlic, leeks, broccoli, rocket (a green leaf), eggs, onions, and scallions.

Chelation Methods

> ➢ Far infrared sauna

> ➢ Sweat inducing exercise

> ➢ Foot ionizing detoxification

> ➢ Activated clay supplements

> ➢ Natural oral chelators

> ➢ IV chelation therapy (adults only)

> ➢ Foods that remove or reduce heavy metals

Natural Oral Chelators

- Cilantro
- Garlic
- Chlorella
- Milk thistle extract
- Alpha lipoic acid
- Organic green barley
- Organic wheatgrass
- Selenium
- Vitamin C
- Vitamin E
- Malic acid
- MSM
- Vitamin B12
- Coenzyme Q10

Orthomolecular Medicine

- NAC (N-Acetyl-L-Cysteine)
- L-carnosine (liquid form, if available)
- L-glutamine
- Taurine
- Lysine
- DL methionine

Nambudripad's Allergy Elimination Techniques (NAET)

A NAET research trial was conducted for young children with autism over a one-year period. The group of children, ages five to seven, was treated with NAET, and the results were remarkable. Verbal skill and physical behavior dramatically improved for many of the children. It did not work on all the children. NAET will require two treatments per week, and the treatments will last approximately thirty-five to forty-five minutes over a period of approximately one year. The severity of the case and the age of the patient will impact recovery time. Nambudripad's Allergy Elimination Technique (NAET) is a technique that eliminates allergies of all types and levels using a blend of medical therapies taken from acupuncture or acupressure, allopathy, chiropractic, nutrition, and kinesiology. It can be noninvasive when acupressure is utilized. It is pain-free, but there may be the presentation of allergic symptoms during the twenty-five hour period following the treatment. The patient needs to be rested, hydrated, and not hungry in order for an optimal treatment. There often is an avoidance period of twenty-five hours after the treatment, where specific items need to be avoided. These items or foods will be identified for the patient at the time of treatment.

One allergen is treated at a time. If the child is not severely immune deficient, he may need just one treatment to desensitize one allergen. Someone with a mild to moderate amount of allergies may take about fifteen to twenty office visits to desensitize fifteen to twenty food and environmental allergens. Basic essential nutrients are treated and cleared during the first few visits. It is important to diagnose and treat the primary allergens that negatively affect the body's ability to maintain health. The longer an allergy goes untreated, the more inflammation occurs. Ordinary items that are not allergens will cause a reaction in a body that is in a state of high inflammation. The inflammation causes swelling, impaired cellular circulation, accelerated aging, and slows cellular detoxification. Extremely ill people with many allergies may require an extended period to get well, but there should be improvement shown after the initial fifteen to twenty treatments.

NAET can be utilized to treat many diseases other than autism, including brain illnesses, cancer, autoimmune diseases, and diabetes. Diseases improve when NAET is used to reduce allergic inflammation throughout the body. Chronic illness usually requires more treatments to produce desired results. Acute situations, such as food poisoning, can respond within two hours. The website to locate a trained NAET practitioner anywhere in the world is www.naet.com.

Melatonin for Sleep Issues in Autism

Sleep problems are reported in most autism children. A clinical research study performed by the Medical Investigation of Neurodevelopmental Disorders (MIND) Institute at the University of California Davis Health System in Sacramento used three milligrams of melatonin at bedtime to treat sleep problems in autistic children. The small study showed improvement in sleep durations and the time children fell asleep.

Herbs

> Ginkgo biloba

- ➢ Valerian root

- ➢ Lemon balm

- ➢ Passionflower

- ➢ Lavender

- ➢ Rooibos (African)

- ➢ Nettle

- ➢ Chamomile (German)

- ➢ Skullcap (Cherokee)

- ➢ St. John's wort

Secretin Hormone Therapy

There are many theories on a gut/brain connection in medicine. Research clinical studies have used the hormone secretin to treat many diseases. Secretin is a hormone that is a peptide that regulates the pH of the intestine through secretion of gastic or stomach acid. Secretin production is impacted by the connection between brain dysfunction and gastrointestinal disorders. As secretin levels rise, the amount of bile secreted by the liver increases. Secretin may affect the anger level of a child with autism due improved liver and pancreas function. The health of the liver is directly connected to its ability to process hormones and detoxify drugs from the body. Increases in levels of bile may allow the body to more quickly detoxify and remove toxins in the liver. This would include chemicals that are found in processed foods or contaminated water. Autism is one type of brain dysfunction that can change secretin levels in children.[1]

Secretin can manage glucose spikes levels by stimulating the pancreas to release more insulin hormone.[2] Secretin also is one of the body's tools to moderate inflammation. Maintaining relatively constant blood glucose levels helps suppress inflammation. Glucose inflammation occurs throughout the body, including the brain. The brain dysfunction associated with autism is negatively impacted by high blood glucose levels. More information on secretin may be found online in Wikipedia.

Secretin has been used experimentally on over one hundred children, but a small clinical research study on three children is the only study published. These three children with autism

---

[1]   United States National Institutes of Health, "The Use of Secretin to Treat Autism," NIH News Alert (10-16-1998).

[2]   http://www.vivo.colostate.edu/hbooks/pathphys/endocrine/gi/secretin.html

received intravenous administration of secretin to stimulate pancreaticobiliary secretion. The secretin IV produced a very significant reduction of gastro-intestinal produced symptoms and caused a large improvement in the children's eye contact, alertness, and expansion of expressive language. These clinical observations suggest an association between gastrointestinal and brain function in patients with autistic behavior.[3] This therapy improves some symptoms in approximately 75 percent of patients, but it is not a cure.

Oxytocin Hormone Therapy

Oxytocin is a hormone and neurotransmitter produced by the anterior lobe of the pituitary. This hormone is associated with the ability to maintain healthy interpersonal relationships and healthy psychological boundaries with other people. If oxytocin levels are abnormal, diagnostic testing for all the hormones produced by the pituitary gland is recommended. It is a hormone that may be lower than normal in those with autism. The disease or symptoms may improve for some when the oxytocin levels increase to the normal range. Autism could raise the required amount of this hormone for this group of patients. In other words, having autism could produce a human body that needs a higher level of this hormone than normal.

University of California, San Diego, researchers theorize that oxytocin acts on the brains of patients with schizophrenia, autism, anxiety, and other brain disorders. It probably increases the level of trust or emotional contact between patient and others. Autistic or schizophrenic patients may lack good eye-to-eye contact with others, focus on less relevant areas of the face, and lack good social interaction.[4] Research has demonstrated that intranasal oxytocin administration reduces stimulation of brain circuits involved in fear, increase levels of eye contact, and increases both trust and generosity. Patients receiving oxytocin hormone do not notice feeling different, but they have altered responses and reactions.

A research study conducted in 1998 discovered that autistic children have significantly lower oxytocin blood plasma levels.[5] A 2007 research study found that oxytocin allowed autistic adults to retain the ability to evaluate the emotional significance of speech intonation.[6]

[3]   K. Horvath, G. Stefanatos, K. N. Sokolski, R. Wachtel, L. Nabors, and J. T. Tildon, "Improved social and language skills after secretin administration in patients with autistic spectrum disorders"," Journal of the Association for Academic Minority Physicians (Sept 1998): 9–15.

[4]   http://www.news-medical.net/news/35124.aspx

[5]   Modahl C, Green L, Fein D et al. (1998). "Plasma oxytocin levels in autistic children". Biol Psychiatry 43 (4): 270–7. doi:0.1016/S0006-3223(97)00439-3. PMID 9513736

[6]   Hollander E, Bartz J, Chaplin W et al. (2007). "Oxytocin increases retention of social cognition in autism". Biol Psychiatry 61 (4): 498–503. doi:10.1016/j.biopsych.2006.05.030. PMID 16904652

Oxytocin reduces cocaine, morphine, heroin, and sweets cravings in animals. When the scientist team managed by Kovacs administered it to rodents that were addicted to cocaine, morphine, or heroin, the rats opted for less of the drugs or showed fewer symptoms of withdrawal.[7] Oxytocin also reduces cravings for sweets.[8] Oxytocin inhibits the development of tolerance to opiates, cocaine, and alcohol and reduces withdrawal symptoms in animal studies.[9] Oxytocin hormone therapy is very new and should be pursued with caution. Most of the research has been on animals. Do not travel overseas for more aggressive treatment with this therapy. Find an experienced research health care professional with this specific area of expertise and associated with a major medical institution.

Research by Dr. E. Hollander suggests the hormone administered intravenously has a positive effect in reducing repetitive behaviors in autism children. Dr. Larry J. Young with the department of psychiatry at Emory University in Atlanta has documented the anti-anxiety effect of oxytocin in small animals. Central administration of oxytocin can impair some learning and memory functions. This should be done in a very closely monitored clinical situation where the doctor is very experienced in this technique.

Fungal Infections in Autistic Children

The gut/brain connection theory extends to autistic symptoms that are made worse by the overgrowth of the Candida albicans fungus. The impaired digestive tract may be due to leaky-gut syndrome, which created an environment for the fungal infection to thrive.

Leaky-gut theory is based upon excess allergens, impaired cellular wall protection, and yeast overgrowth. After the allergies and candida are treated, amino acid therapy should be used to repair the intestinal tract. Probiotics can be utilized to reestablish the beneficial bacteria in the gut after it has been repaired with amino acids. Many autistic children were exposed to large quantities of antibiotics, which can kill the beneficial bacteria and allow candida to thrive. Candida overgrowth also might be caused by hormone treatments, immunosuppressants, herpes virus, chicken pox, high-sugar diets, and chemical exposure.

Removing sugar and sugar replacements from the diet is important in controlling fungal infections. Candida or yeast increases at a much faster rate when exposed to sugar. Antifungal medications like Diflucan, ketoconazole, or Nizoral will eliminate most yeast within one to two months. It usually takes about seven to fourteen days for the yeast to die off; then symptoms can improve significantly. Continued antifungal therapy may be necessary to prevent candida from reestablishing itself. Severe cases of candida have been linked to

[7]

[8] Billings, 2006.

[9] Kovacs GL, Sarnyai Z, Szabo G. (1998) Oxytocin and addiction: a review. Psychoneuroendocrinology 23:945-62 PMID 9924746

autism, schizophrenia, and major depression. Controlling candida is not a cure for autism, but it may significantly reduce the symptoms and improve the health of the patient.

Nutritional supplements and herbs that can reduce candida levels include acidophilus, caprylic acid, garlic oil, olive leaf extract, grapefruit seed extract, Pau D'Arco, propolis, black walnut, germanium, spirulina, skullcap, lemon grass, cinnamon, goldenseal, neem, cat's claw, oregano extract, and colloidal silver.

Dr. William Shaw, author of *Biological Treatments for Autism and PDD*, has been conducting important research on yeast and its effects on autistic individuals. He recently discovered unusual microbial metabolites in the urine of autistic children who responded remarkably well to anti-fungal treatments. Dr. Shaw and his colleagues observed a decrease in urinary organic acids, as well as decreases in hyperactivity and self-stimulatory, stereotyped behavior, and increases in eye contact, vocalization, and concentration.

Music Therapy

Music therapy may help autistic children in many areas, including improvement in social skills, physical coordination when playing an instrument, and enhanced auditory function when singing or playing a harp, piano, or flute. Singing also improves language skills and creativity. Brain-wave activity is enhanced by all types of music therapy. Autistic children may have a tendency to withdraw or shy away from physical contact or interaction. Any activity that children enjoy and that they desire will encourage social interaction. Activity that allows a child to express his or her emotions and joy will accelerate progress in brain development. The vibratory nature of music will impact the body on a cellular level, and singing changes the body's vibration very quickly to that of the music sung or played. The different instruments impact the brain and body in specific ways. A music therapist is trained to utilize this action to improve specific symptoms in autism. This is not an overnight cure, but results have been clinically proven. Music therapy is able to reduce echolalia, the repetitive and uncontrolled use of words.

Animal Therapy

Many types of animal therapy have helped children with brain dysfunction. Animal therapy includes horseback riding, swimming with dolphins, and helping train dogs. This therapy improves the coordination and motor skills of the patient, as well as the emotional well-being. Dolphin therapy has been used for over thirty years. Studies done for the Autism Society have demonstrated that children with disabilities learned faster and retained information longer when they were with dolphins. Violent behavior in autistic children who receive animal therapy is significantly reduced or eliminated.[10] Animal therapy increases decision-making ability and

---

[10] http://ezinearticles.com/?The-Benefits-of-Animal-Therapy-For-Autism&id=1366789

self-confidence in autistic children. This concept can be extended to allowing autistic children to help with farm animals in a supervised manner on a farm or ranch.

Altering Brain-Wave Activity

Hemi Sync is a technique that uses sound to affect brain wave activity. It can be used at home and without a doctor. Hemi-Sync, by the Monroe Institute, uses binaural beating, a sensory-information stimulus, and changes the information sent to the reticular-thalamic activating system, which improves attention, focus, and level of awareness.[11] Hemi-Sync signals contribute to a greater balance of activity between the right and left hemispheres and cortical and subcortical areas of the brain.[12] Hemi-Sync can be used to improve Asperger's syndrome and autism. Children can maximize brain function using Hemi-Sync. It is great for calming children down who have severe behavioral issues through changing brain-wave activity. This technique is very affordable and should be tried for difficult cases to shift the tipping point for this disease.

Cranial electrostimulation (CES) is another way to treat Asperger's and autism. One of its functions is altering brain-wave activity. It enhances neurotransmitter levels and energy production.

Hyperbaric Oxygen Therapy

A small clinical trial was conducted by Dr. Daniel A. Rossini with the International Child Development Resource Center in Melbourne, Florida using hyperbaric oxygen therapy to treat autism. His clinical trial found improvement in the children's language ability, eye contact, and social interaction. Eighty percent of hyperbaric-treated children had improved symptoms.

The treatments proved most beneficial to children over the age of five and patients with less severe autism. There were no side effects from the hyperbaric oxygen therapy.

Auricular Acupuncture for Autism

Auricular acupuncture points utilized:

> - Kidney
> - Heart

---

[11]   http://www.monroeinstitute.org/wiki/index.php/Main_Page

[12]   http://www.incrediblehorizons.com/hemi-sync- education.htm#DEVELOPMENTAL%20DISABILITIES

- Spleen
- Occiput
- Shen men
- Subcortex
- Brain
- Neurasthenia
- Sympathetic

Chinese diagnosis: Autism may be caused by phlegm misting the mind, kidney essence deficiency, blood and qi deficiency with blood stagnation, and blood heat from toxins.

Interactive Metronome (IM) Therapy

Interactive metronome (IM) therapy was created to improve learning and developmental disorders in children. It is also effective for adults in brain rehabilitation. IM is a neuromotor assessment and treatment tool that is used to improve the neurological processes of motor planning and sequencing. IM improves motor planning and sequencing by using neurosensory and neuromotor exercises to increase brain plasticity.

The human brain's efficiency and performance depend on the seamless transition of neuron network signals from one area of the brain to another. The research of Neal Alpine, MD, suggests that IM works by augmenting the internal-processing speed within the neuroaxis. The brain is affected in the cerebellum, prefrontal cortex, cingulate gyrus, and basal ganglia. This area is responsible for sustained attention, language formulation, motor coordination, and balance.

The IM program provides a structured, goal-oriented process that challenges the patient to synchronize a range of hand and foot exercises to a precise computer-generated reference tone heard through headphones. IM requires a series of twelve to fifteen sessions. It works through listening through stereo headphones to a rhythmic sound and responding by tapping or clapping and attempting to match the beat. A patented auditory-visual guidance system provides immediate feedback measured in milliseconds, and a score is provided.[13]

IM trains the brain to learn rhythm and timing. As timing improves, so do motor control,

---

[13]   http://www.interactivemetronome.com/IMPublic/Home.aspx

coordination, focus, concentration, language processing, aggression, impulsiveness, endurance, strength, filtering out distractions, attention span, self-control, school performance, and social performance. IM has been used to treat dyslexia, sensory integration disorder, ADHD, traumatic brain injury (TBI), cerebral vascular accident (CVA), autism spectrum disorder, cerebral palsy, non-verbal learning disorder, Asperger's syndrome, delayed speech development, Parkinson's disease, and balance problems.[14]

IM research is currently being conducted at the following institutions:

- ➤ Drexel University is working on durability and generalization

- ➤ University of Rochester is working on visual attention

- ➤ University of Cincinnati studied hemiplegic arm

- ➤ Medical College of Georgia researched Parkinson's disease

- ➤ Veterans Administration researched cognitive, behavioral and motor skills (unimpaired and veterans with blast injuries)

- ➤ Walter Reed Army Medical Center studied PTSD, sleep, and cognitive

Applied Behavior Analysis (ABA)

Applied behavior analysis (ABA) uses behavior to improve social skills and change previous behavior patterns. ABA must be applied, behavioral, analytic, technological, conceptually systematic, and effective.[15]

Behaviors are characterized in observable and measurable terms in order to determine change over time.[16] The behavior is analyzed in a given environment to detect all the specific factors that are influencing the behavior.

After an initial assessment is completed, identifying the specific skills of each patient, treatment goals are chosen for the patient. These goals are set using the initial assessment information. This is broken down further into the curriculum scope and sequence that lists skills in all domains, including learning, communication, social, academic, self-care, motor, play, and leisure. The goals are divided into smaller component skills from simple to complex. The goal is to help the patient to develop skills to allow him to function independently and

---

[14] http://www.akcsm.com/services_IM.htm

[15] DONALD M. BAER, MONTROSE M. WOLF, AND TODD R. RISLEY SOME CURRENT DIMENSIONS OF APPLIED BEHAVIOR ANALYSIS' JOURNAL OF APPLIED BEHAVIOR ANALYSIS. 1968, 1, 91-97

[16] http://en.wikipedia.org/wiki/Applied_behavior_analysis#cite_note-As-in-ABA-14

successfully.[17]

ABA-based interventions are used to treat people with a wide variety of behaviors and diagnoses, notably autism spectrum disorders,[18] as well as in ABA is utilized in treating schizophrenia.[19] It can also be used to treat severe mental disorders, learning language, disease prevention, conservation of electricity, prevention of littering, and more.

Auditory Integration Training (AIT)

Distortions in hearing or auditory processing in the brain contribute to behavioral or learning disorders, such as autism spectrum disorder. Auditory integration training (AIT) is a controversial therapy but may be useful in treating autism spectrum disorder, as well as dyslexia, anxiety, depression, ADD, ADHD, central auditory processing disorders (CAPD), speech disorders, sensory disorders, and pervasive developmental disorder (PDD).[20] This therapy will not work for many people, but where hearing problems have the largest impact on the patient, it could be extremely useful.

AIT may help in correcting or improving auditory processing problems that may occur if the auditory messages received by the brain are distorted. If an individual's hearing ability is different between the two ears, it results in sounds being perceived in an extremely different way. AIT works to normalize the hearing of both ears. It is also used for hypersensitivity to sound.

AIT requires listening to vocal music through headphones connected to an electronic device that electronically transforms the sounds. These sessions last about thirty minutes, typically twice a day for ten consecutive days. Before receiving the AIT, the individual is given an audiogram to determine the hearing ability for various sound frequencies. After this, the individual listens to music through a special machine through the earphones.

Osteopathic Manipulation

Osteopathic manipulation was done in a clinical research study of twenty-five children. This

---

17 http://www.behavior.org/autism/

18 Dillenburger K, Keenan M (2009). "None of the As in ABA stand for autism: dispelling the myths". *J Intellect Dev Disabil* **34** (2): 193–5. doi:10.1080/13668250902845244. PMID

19 Wong, S. E., Martinez-Diaz, J. A., Massel, H. K., Edelstein, B. A., Wiegand, W., Bowen, L., & Liberman, R. P. (1993). Conversational skills training with schizophrenic inpatients: A study of generalization across settings and conversants. Behavior Therapy, 24, 285-304.

20 http://www.aithelps.com/

therapy involves moving bones which affects muscles and nerves of the child. Almost all of the children had received additional alternative therapies of some type. Twenty-two of the children exhibited a common cranial distortion. This distortion was compression and/or restriction of the left middle cranial fascia, with an overlying hyperflexion type of pattern at the spheno-basilar synthesis. This compression impaired the central nervous system. After treatment, fifteen of the children were communicating in sentences of four words or more, initiating social contact, and demonstrating spontaneous imaginative play. A single child was fully recovered. Eleven children were in regular preschool, kindergarten, or grade school with limited assistance. Thirteen children were in special school programs for autistic children. This therapy works well on three-year-old children but can also be useful in children ages four and five.[21]

---

[21] http://www.studentdoctor.net/blogs/omtguru/2006/03/osteopathic-medicine-and-autism.html

DEPRESSION

Depression can be a life-threatening illness or one that can be treated without medication for those fortunate enough to have a doctor familiar with alternative medicine. The symptoms can include weight gain, sloppiness, arriving late for work, failure to shower, not wearing makeup for some women, insomnia, sleeping too long, brain fog, not taking care of one's appearance, excessive drinking, and an increase in recreational drug use.

External factors like job loss, death, financial loss, and natural disasters can trigger depression. Internal causes can be related to hormone imbalances, mineral deficiencies, imbalances of vitamin levels, poor diet, low dietary enzymes, and allergies. Medicines such as antibiotics, cocaine, heroin, crystal meth, barbiturates, amphetamines, painkillers, beta-blockers, anti-Parkinson's drugs, blood pressure drugs, heart medications, and psychotropic drugs may cause or contribute to depression, stress, anxiety, and bipolar disorder. Any medicine reducing the level of your hormones can cause depression or bipolar disorder.

The brain can be stimulated with several types of outside energy, including magnetic therapy, implanted electrodes for electrical stimulation, and laser therapy. The development of new medical products that heal or treat depression continues to increase. These therapies may work well in deficient-type patients. Depression accompanied by severe pain must be treated separately. It is always important to look to secondary illnesses that might accompany depression, including herpes, diabetes, MS, Alzheimer's, Parkinson's, and brain tumors. Your health care provider should not ever treat your depression without a full set of diagnostic tests.

Depression may benefit from many types of alternative medical therapies. Several factors influence the doctor's depression therapy of choice. These factors include the length of time the patient has suffered from depression, as well as the patient's age, dietary habits, and use of natural supplements.

It is better to treat depression with a comprehensive treatment plan of nutritional support, exercise, dietary changes, and amino acid therapy. A person with severe depression will require laser acupuncture and amino acid therapy or Chinese herbal formulas. The use of three therapies together can transform even the most severe depression for most people. The addition of an affordable medical device called the Alpha-Stim 100, which uses microcurrent electrical therapy, will complete the best of Quantum Brain Healing's suggested top cures and treatments for depression. The Alpha-Stim 100 is available through doctors, chiropractors, or acupuncturists.

Depression may return under extreme circumstances and can be treated more quickly the second time due to the information accumulated when treating the initial event. A causative factor for depression may be inadequate or interrupted sleep. If there is a melatonin deficiency, the body's circadian rhythm is imbalanced, and the body will wake up at irregular times due to brain-wave irregularities and hormone imbalances. Bach Flower Remedies and aromatherapy can help most people gently fall asleep. Try lavender aromatherapy to fall asleep and orange aromatherapy to wake up. Bergamot aromatherapy is extremely good for those with depression. When you have depression, put several drops of bergamot oil on your pillowcase and on your face.

Depression is a multifaceted disease that should be analyzed early for organic causes. Hormones imbalances should be tested, and blood work should be evaluated for bacterial or viral infections. Hormone imbalances can be corrected with Chinese herbal patent formulas like Xiao Yao Wan, Jia Wei Xiao Yao Wan, Shui De, Gui Pi Tang, Gan Mai Da Zao Tang, and Chai Hu Shu Gan San.

Chinese patent formulas will take approximately two to five weeks for the full extent of their benefits to be viewed relative to hormone changes. Depression can lift of its own accord when hormone issues are managed.

Diet

The diet for depression should include fresh cold-water fish, such as mackerel, eaten several times per week. The diet should be high in unsaturated fats and may include snacks of walnuts and almonds. The cell membrane of your neuron contains a small amount omega-3. Higher amounts of omega-3 levels could make a more stable and flexible cell membrane so that serotonin or dopamine remain in the cell longer. Purified fish oil may extend the life of serotonin, as vitamins E and C can extend the life of other antioxidants. Fish oil has direct effects on neurotransmitter levels. This impacts bipolar disorder and depression prognoses. Other foods like salmon, mackerel, avocado, and walnuts are high in omega-3 essential fatty acids and enhance for brain health.

Try to reduce or eliminate food additives, artificial sweeteners, high-fructose corn syrup, alcohol, nicotine, nitrates, refined foods, and food dyes. The diet should eliminate genetically modified foods and should include organic fruits and vegetables. A food-based multivitamin should be taken on a daily basis. One to two cups of Earl Gray tea per day may help many people with depression - it contains bergamot. Reduce your consumption of breads and pasta. It is important for your daily protein level to be sufficient. Whey or rice protein can be taken for breakfast or as a snack food to increase your protein levels. People with depression may improve with a diet low in refined sugar. Stevia, molasses, maple syrup, and turbinado sugar are better choices as sweeteners.

Insomnia Related to Depression

The use of a very inexpensive melatonin supplement - 1.5 to 3 mg/d for approximately four weeks - could help this type of deficiency. Another sleep aid is a combination capsule containing vitamin D, magnesium, and calcium. Several herbs which can help a person improve sleep, including St. John's wort, hops, valerian, passionflower, chamomile, and lemon balm. Bach Flower Remedies are a wonderful, mild tool for helping people relax; they also can treat depression and insomnia. Aromatic essential oils also are a great tool. There are small pillows filled with lavender that can be warmed in the microwave to release the aroma. This might be the very idea to try for an elderly patient. Orthomolecular Medicine can also be used to treat insomnia.

Vitamins

Quantum Brain Healing uses vitamin B12 is as a way to improve the brain in several ways. Vitamin B12 is involved in DNA synthesis and fatty acid synthesis. It helps break down carbohydrates and covert them into energy. It is used by the body to help make several amino acids, including SAM-e. These amino acids change brain chemistry and neurotransmitter levels. The neurotransmitters affected by vitamin B12 directly are involved in learning skills and memory. Vitamin B12 is found in beef, caviar, chicken, cheese, eggs, fish, lamb, liver, milk, octopus, and shellfish. A sublingual form of this vitamin is available. A multivitamin product should also be taken with this supplement so that the other B vitamins do not become deficient.

Symptoms of vitamin B12 deficiency include depression, fatigue, brain fog, delusion, poor memory, neurological problems, poor concentration, psychosis, irritability, mania, forgetfulness, and increased sleep requirements. These symptoms may also be indicative of other vitamin or mineral deficiencies. Any of these conditions may be treated with this vitamin if a deficiency exists. Many people have multiple vitamin deficiencies. They all must be treated for the patient to heal.

Quantum Orthomolecular Medicine uses higher amounts of vitamin B12 than would be found in multivitamin product or normal diet. Many brain diseases may require these higher levels of vitamin B12 in order for healing to occur. Diseases improved by taking vitamin B12 include depression, Alzheimer's disease, dementia, long-term memory loss, and impaired ability to convert short-term memory into long-term memory. The brain fog symptom associated with chronic fatigue syndrome can be improved with increased doses of this supplement. It is always worth noting that digestive problems may be the root of vitamin deficiencies. A digestive enzyme may allow you to better absorb most of your vitamins.

Coenzyme Q10, or CoQ10, is a ubiquinone and a cofactor in energy production. It is a coenzyme used in energy production by the mitochondria. CoQ10 affects many neurological functions. It is best taken with food that contains some type of lipid or fat—this increase energy production and improve serious fatigue. Take this with 1500 mg per day malic acid for chronic fatigue syndrome or any extreme case of fatigue that is not due to viral or bacterial infection.

Choline is brain food. CDP-choline is a form of choline and cytidine. Choline is a precursor to phosphatidylcholine (PS). It is used in the structure and function of cells. It is a precursor to acetylcholine. CDP-choline can affect many neurological functions. Its actions include crossing blood-brain barrier. It improves immune and cognitive function for those with PTSD. It improves neurological function in an overstressed person and protects the brain. It helps balance the brain and this action improves depression.

Vitamin C can be taken in large amounts to act as an antioxidant and detoxification agent. It will help your body fight stress and support your immune system. It is found in kiwi, oranges, lemons, cantaloupes, cherries, and many other fruits.

Minerals

Boron can help prevent depression. Boron is a trace mineral and functions as an activation agent and coenzyme in your body's metabolism. This trace mineral helps regulate the levels of calcium, magnesium, and phosphorus. You can find boron in apples, avocados, grapes, legumes, nuts, pears, plums, prunes, raisins, and tomatoes. Boron is an antioxidant and is a key anti-aging trace mineral. The most important use of boron in your body is to prevent and reduce inflammation throughout the body. It also is important in helping the body fight viral infections by increasing the strength of the immune system.

Boron is involved in Quantum Brain Healing by its impact on hormone regulation. Boron affects estrogen and testosterone, which are very key hormones in memory and cognitive thinking. These hormone deficiencies may be associated with depression. It is involved in mental alertness, manual dexterity, hand-to-eye coordination, attention, perception, short-term memory, and long-term memory. Boron is very important in treating many brain diseases, including depression, stress, memory difficulties, and cognitive impairment.

Quantum Brain Healing requires the addition of this trace mineral as a supplement. A high-quality supplement may be found in food-based vitamin and mineral products. Treating diseases with Orthomolecular Medicine usually requires higher levels of a substance than are found in most vitamin supplements or in foods. Diseases frequently increase the level of a vitamin or mineral needed in the body to maintain good health. The RDA of vitamins and minerals is not sufficient for those suffering from serious illness or health issues.

Intravenous Therapy or Myers Cocktail

The Myers Cocktail is an intravenous therapy consisting of mixes of vitamins, minerals, amino acids, and other nutrients. It can be very useful in treating emotional issues due to fatigue and overexertion. Depression due to nutritional deficiencies can resolve itself very quickly after a course of IV vitamins and minerals. You can feel the results within twenty-four hours. When nutrients are given intravenously, your digestive system is bypassed and a much higher level of nutrition can be delivered directly to your cells via the bloodstream. Dr. John Myers was the first doctor to develop an intravenous nutrient therapy that obtained positive clinical results for a variety of medical conditions. This is alternative medicine at its best.

The Myers Cocktail improves almost all digestive symptoms, including bloating, diarrhea, food allergies, irritable bowel syndrome, colitis, ulcers, and Crohn's disease. Depression can stem from B-vitamin deficiencies.

The Myers Cocktail intravenous therapy improves the body's ability to make energy and increases cellular function. You may feel a warm sensation while the IV is administered. The effect is usually fast, but extremely ill people will require several treatments to experience the full effect.

The Myers Cocktail IV therapy may be helpful for chronic or acute conditions, including digestive problems, mental fatigue, PTSD, fatigue, fibromyalgia, depression, bacterial or viral infection, asthma, cardiac pain, congestive heart failure, palpitations, migraine headaches, cardiovascular disease, respiratory problems, seasonal allergies, hives, hyperthyroidism, and muscle spasms due to nutritional deficiency.

Nutritional Supplements

Quantum Brain Healing uses melatonin to help treat depression, along with amino acids, vitamins, minerals, and herbs. Melatonin is a hormone produced in the brain by the pineal gland from the amino acid tryptophan. It is available as a nutritional supplement. You can also increase melatonin levels by supplementing the amino acid tryptophan. Melatonin is stimulated by darkness and suppressed by light, and it is affected by the circadian rhythm. It regulates diverse body functions. Levels of melatonin in the blood are highest prior to bedtime. Low levels of melatonin are associated with some types of cancer.

Melatonin will help treat depression that stems from inadequate sleep. When the sleep cycle is improved, this type of depression patient often will recover quickly. Anxiety is also a problem when there is sleep deprivation. Almost every type of brain condition gets worse when there is insufficient sleep. It is important to ask your doctor how to resolve this problem.

Hormone imbalances often cause many brain conditions during menopause or andropause (male menopause).

Melatonin will cross the blood-brain barrier to increase brain circulation and increase the production of neurotransmitters to balance the brain. It strengthens the immune system. The enhanced immune system is due to the improvement in hormone and neurotransmitter regulation.

DHEA is a natural hormone precursor to estrogen and androgen produced from cholesterol. Your body's own DHEA levels may be reduced by taking insulin, corticosteroids, opiates, or danazol. It affects the cortex of the brain. DHEA can lower the levels of interleukin-6 to affect your immune system. DHEA affects the brain to improve mood and acts as an anti-inflammatory and immunity enhancer. The increase in DHEA level may directly improve depression.

Quantum Brain Healing uses melatonin to treat insomnia, jet lag, ischemia, smoking cessation, sleep disturbances related to depression, depression caused by sleep deprivation, seasonal affective disorder (SAD), and anxiety. This hormone may be combined with amino acids to increase its effectiveness. Nutritional support can include food-based multivitamins, vitamin E, vitamin D, CoQ10, and alpha lipoic acid.

Amino Acid Therapy

Quantum Brain Healing also uses amino acids to improve brain chemistry and balance neurotransmitter levels. The amino acids used include 5-HTP, SAM-e, GABA, and tyrosine. Amino acids may have to be combined for many people, while other people may be able to use a single amino acid to turn around their depression.

It is extremely important to understand that smoking, recreational drugs, and alcohol contribute to significant increases in depression. Cigarette smokers are 41 percent more likely to suffer from depression than nonsmokers. Smoking a pipe or cigar also increases depression. Smoking cessation of all types is important to resolving depression. The increased carbon monoxide levels from cigarette smoking probably impact the increased depression levels.

Amino acid therapy for depression is a wonderful option for teenagers. This is a healthy alternative as the drugs for depression have not been tested on children and teenagers. Most children do not need treatment for depression. They need lifestyle changes, including more exercise and less refined foods in their diets. The elimination of carbonated beverages and high fructose will improve the moods of many children.

GABA is an amino acid used in the field of holistic healing to treat depression, insomnia, and anxiety. It may be very effective for those people who cannot use antidepressants due to side effects. GABA is an amino acid that is a calming neurotransmitter, and it is usually deficient in those with depression and anxiety. GABA may also be useful in treating OCD and insomnia. Several neurotransmitters frequently are imbalanced in most brain diseases.

Quantum Brain Healing can treat several addictions with Orthomolecular Medicine. It focus on using amino acid therapy and antioxidants supplements to heal the brain. Amino acid therapy can help addicts recover from valium, pot, alcohol, and food additives.

Using GABA for addiction issues should be a long-term strategy. This supplement should be added for two to five years. Valium addiction frequently occurs due to severe anxiety when the patient is attempting to self-treat anxiety or depression. GABA is not effective in treating severe depression or bipolar disorder.

Another amino acid that is used in Orthomolecular Medicine is 5-HTP. This supplement can be used in mild cases of neuropathy to calm overstimulated or overexcited nerves. This amino acid also can replace tricyclic antidepressants used in the treatment of neuropathy, in some cases. 5-HTP may be used at higher doses to treat overeating related to mood disorders and depression in a mild to moderate case. Extremely severe cases may not be able to use this treatment protocol to replace drug therapy, but it may be useful in serious cases to lower the amount of the drug required by the patient.

Depression can often be abated within a two-to-four week period by taking 5-HTP at doses of 50–300 mg three times a day. The dosage is dependent on the weight, size, age, and physical condition of the person. The 5-HTP increases the body's serotonin level; it may be taken with food. Any insomnia associated with the depression may improve significantly. 5-HTP may not work for everyone and may cause slight nausea. Do not use 5-HTP in combination with drugs that increase serotonin (SRRIs).

SAM-e is another amino acid that will work alone for many people to resolve depression within two to three weeks. Try taking 400 mg of SAM-e before bed on an empty stomach as an effective way to resolve depression. SAM-e should be taken for four to six weeks before deciding on its effectiveness.

Trace Mineral Salts

Quantum Brain Healing utilizes lithium orotate to repair RNA and DNA. This trace mineral salt can travel inside the brain and stabilize many of the chemical activities of the neurons or brain cells. It is a neuron protectant and protects brain cells in the hippocampus, striatum, and frontal cortex of the brain. It helps support neural plasticity and helps reduce mental stress. It stimulates the growth of new neurons.

Lithium orotate can stimulate the repair of damaged nerve tissue. If you are using lithium orotate, it is important to include other nutrients in therapeutic doses for a least one year. Alpha lipoic acid should be used at a level of 200 to 600 mg per day for this purpose. Use a good food-based multivitamin on a daily basis to help your body fully utilize any trace mineral and mineral salt. This helps balance neurotransmitter levels for those with depression and several substance abuse-type illnesses.

Lithium orotate is very effective for moderate to severe depression that does not respond to drugs. The moderately serious depression patient may also need to add therapeutic doses of amino acids. The levels of supplements will have to be monitored very closely, for it is difficult to predict the exact amounts needed of this trace mineral salt and how it reacts with the amino acids. Brain metabolism for very seriously ill people is a challenge for any doctor to predict. Tea made with rose hips is good for those who are severely depressed. Rose hips are a very good source of antioxidants. Bipolar disorder also can be treated with this trace mineral salt.

Evaluating the sleep environment and removing allergens is often helpful for alleviating depression. Remove feather pillows, and use cotton, silk, or wool products on the bed. An air ionizing machine from Sharper Image can improve air-quality issues. You also might invest in an ionizing filtration system for the air conditioning and heating unit for the entire household. Sleep may be interrupted due to the temperature of the air. The successful management of insomnia can go a very long way in treating depression.

The use of sunlight has long been an inexpensive and exceptional way to treat mild depression, when combined with moderate exercise four to five days per week. The Sharper Image offers a sunlamp that artificially provides sunlight. Patients should be cautious about the recent trend to replace full-spectrum lighting with energy-saving fluorescent lighting, as this can make depression worse for some patients. This could occur in homes without many outside windows or where the windows are always covered. Depression or seasonal affective disorder (SAD) can be triggered in many northern climates during the winter, particularly by those who are prone to depression. The inclusion of liquid vitamin D3 and calcium supplements on a regular basis can help these people.

NAET

Nambudripad's Allergy Elimination Technique (NAET) eliminates allergies of all types and levels, using a blend of medical therapies taken from acupuncture or acupressure, allopathy, chiropractic, nutrition, and kinesiology. It can be noninvasive when acupressure is utilized. It is pain-free, but allergic symptoms may present during the twenty-five hour period following the treatment. For an optimal treatment, the patient needs to be rested, hydrated, and not hungry. There is usually an avoidance period of twenty-five hours after the treatment, where specific items need to be avoided. These items or foods will be identified for the patient at the time of treatment.

NAET can be used to treat and improve many brain illnesses. Most diseases are impacted by environmental or food allergies. Depression patients can be treated for allergens. This will help the immune system improve and will improve the patient's prognosis. It does not work on all people. NAET will require about two treatments per week; treatments last approximately thirty-five to forty-five minutes over a period of approximately one year. The severity of the depression and the age of the patient will determine the number of sessions required. Chronic depression takes longer to heal. People with depression would be wise to limit the intake of sugar, vinegar, alcohol, tobacco, genetically modified foods, and sweets.

One allergen is treated at a time. If you are not severely immune deficient, you may need just one treatment to desensitize one allergen. Alzheimer's and Parkinson's patients have immune systems that are under attack. Any additional symptoms such as depression, anxiety, insomnia, memory loss, and alcoholism will require additional attention and treatment. A person with a mild to moderate amount of allergies may take about fifteen to twenty office visits to desensitize fifteen to twenty food and environmental allergens. Basic essential nutrients are treated and cleared during the first few visits. It is important to diagnose and treat the primary allergens that negatively affect the body's ability to maintain health. The longer an allergy goes untreated, the more inflammation occurs. Ordinary items that are not allergens will cause a reaction in a body when it is in a state of high inflammation. Extremely ill people with many allergies may require an extended period to get well, but there should be some improvement shown after the initial fifteen to twenty treatments.

NAET can be utilized to treat many diseases, including depression, insomnia, smoking cessation, concentration problems, brain fog, brain illnesses, and diabetes. Diseases improve when NAET is used to reduce allergenic inflammation throughout the body. Chronic illness usually requires more treatments to produce desired results. Acute situations, such as food poisoning, can respond within two hours. The website to locate a trained NAET practitioner anywhere in the world can be found at www.NAET.com.

Exercise

Many people develop depression from lack of exercise combined with poor diets. Poor diets affect brain chemistry. A diet lacking in adequate unsaturated fats can cause depression-like symptoms. An exercise plan of thirty minutes three times per week for ten weeks can relieve depression as effectively as antidepressants.

Prayer can relieve or reduce depression. An organized prayer group can be effective for cases of difficult depression. A vision of wellness is held while prayer is conducted for the person over a six-month period. Prayer can be an effective way to relieve stress or anxiety for many people. Churches sometimes offer exercise groups and yoga Zen centers may offer meditation and tai chi sessions.

Many doctors will request that the patient include a mild form of exercise such as yoga, gardening, walking, biking, tai chi, qi gong, or volleyball. This is especially true for children suffering from depression. Children with depression should be encouraged to be socially active. Older patients can walk or do mild exercise in their chair.

Chi machines allow patients to lie on the floor and put their legs on to a machine, which will move their legs in a slow motion from side to side. This will improve circulation for patients who may not be able to walk. Swimming can be another option, but it is important to watch for chlorine allergies. It is also important to pay extra attention to the diets of children and older patients. Severe dietary allergies are known to cause depression.

Yoga is extremely beneficial for depression, as it affects the entire endocrine system and reduces cortisol. Practicing qi gong and tai chi can alter hormones and neurotransmitters in the brain. It will take at least two to four times per week of yoga, tai chi, or qi gong to change hormones to the level needed to lift depression. This type of exercise is needed on a long-term basis in order to sustain the results.

Yoga

Yoga is a great way to increase circulation, improve flexibility, reduce stress, balance hormone function, restore proper sleep cycles, and improve energy flow. There are many types of yoga that offer different health benefits.

Power yoga is aerobic in nature and will burn more calories and improve circulation more quickly. It requires that the participant be healthy. A yoga posture, or asana, may be repeated quickly several times. There are standing and floor postures. Classes usually last one hour.

Hatha yoga increases balance, flexibility, and fitness at a gentle pace suitable for almost everyone. People of all ages and levels of fitness can do this yoga. It is very important to discuss all health problems with the yoga instructor prior to class so you can be guided in which postures need to be avoided for specific health concerns.

Bikram yoga or "hot yoga" is a great way to detoxify, increase flexibility, and increase metabolism. It is important to take water with you to class. This practice involves performing yoga postures for ninety minutes in a heated room. The first half of the session involves standing postures, while the second half of the class is floor postures. Because muscles are warm, most people are able to increase flexibility at a faster rate. Do not push yourself in this class until you are experienced in how the heat will affect you. Do not do this yoga every day, as it can result in electrolyte imbalances. If you are feeling dizzy after class, replenish your electrolytes with a supplement.

For some people with arthritis or other motion-limiting issues, herbs can improve their yoga practice and take it to the next level. Herbs can increase flexibility, promote circulation, and stimulate the movement of energy. Herbs can aid in the proper performance of postures by improving circulation, joint function, balance, and coordination. They may be referred to as anti-rheumatic or anti-arthritic agents.

They are mainly herbs for Hatha yoga. Hatha yoga is gentle and can benefit from the use of herbs that are not suitable for power or hot yoga or Bikram yoga. Herbs that can be used in this fashion include adaptogenic herbs such as ashwagandha, panax ginseng, and huang qi. Other herbs used to improve circulation or flexibility in people with arthritis or motor-limiting issues include guggul, shallaki, myrrh, nirgundi, turmeric, saffron, curcumin, sage, salvia, Siberian ginseng, green tea, guarana, Bacopa monnieri, ginkgo biloba, angelica, kava kava, and dasha mula.

Yoga is an amazing tool for athletic people to manage chronic pain. Professional athletes often have success in using Bikram yoga to replace strong pain medications for solving chronic pain after the muscle or ligament tears have healed. For some people with arthritis or other motion-limiting issues, herbs can improve their yoga practice and take it to the next level. Herbs can increase flexibility, promote circulation, and stimulate the movement of energy. Herbs can aid in the proper performance of postures by improving circulation, joint function, balance, and coordination. They may be referred to as anti-rheumatic or anti-arthritic agents. Herbs that are adaptogens can help people in their yoga. Contact an herbalist.

Several yoga poses are wonderful for helping balance the body to treat depression, including Downward Facing Dog, Child Pose, Head to Knee Pose, Boat Pose, and Fish Pose.

Qi Gong

Qi gong is an ancient type of Chinese energy work that can transform anyone's health. Qi gong influences electromagnetic energy throughout the body. It can change electrical activity in the body and balance blood flow and cellular water balance. This type of energy work is a slow and controlled movement of the body and its qi. The correct movement by the body can improve its energy. Long-term qi gong will help improve energy levels, improve sleep, and balance hormone and neurotransmitters. It can be done in a group setting or by yourself. It has so many movements that some may be difficult to recall. The use of a DVD can help novices with their qi gong practice. Qi gong is an energy form that has many benefits similar to tai chi, Therapeutic Touch, and Reiki.

The medical benefits of qi gong include increasing brain circulation, lowering or increasing blood pressure levels toward a moderate level, and balancing endocrine gland function. This improves your hormone and neurotransmitter levels and reduces hypertension. This form of ancient Chinese energy work decreases the occurrence of strokes and improves your sex life. It is anti-aging, increases your immune function, and helps manage asthma. People live longer after including a long-term qi gong practice in their lives.

Qi gong increases activity in the prefrontal cortex and amygdala. It increases brain relaxation and reduces stress. It can heal anxiety and sleep disorders and treats mild and moderate depression. It can improve oxygen levels; it improves positive thoughts. It is very helpful for people in recovery from serious diseases like cancer, ischemia, and stroke.

Energy work can reduce the cost of health care. The person without depression or anxiety is less prone to disease because his or her immune system function at a higher level. This form of energy work may be adapted so that it can be performed in a chair - this would be the arm and upper-body movements of qi gong that stimulate and heal the body. It can even be done is a hospital bed.

Herbs

Several Chinese patent formulas can quickly treat depression for many people. Depression is a multifaceted disease that should be analyzed early for organic causes. Hormone imbalances should be tested and blood work should be evaluated for bacterial or viral infections. Chinese patent formulas can treat the underlying root diseases, as well as the depression. Hormone imbalances can result in depression. There are many Chinese herbal patent formulas to treat depression, such as Xiao Yao Wan, Jia Wei Xiao Yao Wan, Shui De, Gui Pi Tang, Gan Mai Da Zao Tang, and Chai Hu Shu Gan San. These affordable herbal products can be obtained through an acupuncturist or herbalist.

Chinese patent formulas will take approximately two-to-five weeks for the full extent of their benefits to be viewed, relative to hormone changes. Depression can lift on its own accord when these issues are managed. Another causative factor for depression may be inadequate or interrupted sleep. If there is a melatonin deficiency, the body's circadian rhythm is imbalanced, and the body will wake up at irregular times due to brainwave irregularities and hormone imbalances.

Many single herbs can treat or heal depression, including ginseng, catuaba, gotu kola, muira puama, ashwagandha, astragalus, Siberian snow rose, valerian, St. John's wort, lemon balm, lemongrass, milk thistle, skullcap, and vinpocetine.

Catuaba is a South American herb that has many medical properties, including the ability to act as an antibiotic and antiviral. It also is an adaptogen and can sedate or stimulate the brain and central nervous system as needed. It is an antioxidant and may be an anti-aging herb for the brain. Catuaba is an analgesic and can calm the brain when overstimulation has occurred.

Catuaba can treat many diseases, including depression, anxiety, poor memory, dementia, stress, fatigue, neuralgia, nervous exhaustion, sciatica, and Alzheimer's disease. Many of these diseases are very closely related. Fatigue, anxiety, stress, depression, and nervous exhaustion may be diseases on a continuum. Early in a cycle, the disease manifested is anxiety, and later, manifestation may be nervous exhaustion or depression.

This herb should not be considered a sole treatment. It should be combined with nutritional supplements, including amino acids. This is not a common herb but will be available to health care professionals. Several herbs are often used for this group of illnesses. Catuaba is one of the secondary herbs to be considered.

A liver detoxification prior to the use of catuaba may improve or hasten its success. Quantum Brain Healing relies on the use of therapeutic minerals and vitamins to rebalance the body. Many of these diseases require large doses of calcium, magnesium and vitamin D to stabilize the sleep cycles of the patients. Irregular sleep cycles usually make diseases worse and impair good health. The key factor of this herb is that it is an adaptogen.

Gotu kola is used to heal or treat many brain diseases, like stress, epilepsy, Alzheimer's disease, mental fatigue, neurasthenia, and even insanity. Gotu kola is also known as ji xue cao in China. Gotu kola has many important actions to help the brain repair itself, including increasing brain circulation and acting as an anti-inflammatory. Gotu kola's ability to enhance brain circulation while reducing inflammation is a major way it treats brain diseases. It is a mild diuretic. Gotu kola is also an anti-inflammatory substance that can reduce or prevent inflammation throughout the body. This herb is an adaptogen, which means it will act to balance the body. It can stimulate or sedate, depending on the action needed by the body for optimal health.

Gotu kola affects neurotransmitter levels in the brain. Herbs can indirectly impact the level of certain neurotransmitters levels, like GABA, in the brain for curing and treating depression and eating disorders. This herb directly affects the cortex of the brain and can target the GABA receptor sites to balance neurotransmitter levels. This is a very effective herbal product.

Muira puama is a highly active herb with many active chemical components. This herb crosses blood-brain barrier and increases circulation in several areas of the brain, including the hippocampus, cerebral cortex, hypothalamus, and cerebellum areas, and the central nervous system. It is an antioxidant that affects the nervous system to improve nerve diseases, including ALS and MS. The herb may have use in treating impaired nerve function due to accident or trauma. For nerve injuries and diseases, Quantum Brain Healing utilizes several supplements, including alpha lipoic acid and high-quality fish oil or cod liver supplements. Diets for nerve injuries and diseases must include high levels of unsaturated fatty acids, B vitamins, and choline.

Muira puama is an adaptogen and can stimulate or sedate, depending on what the person's body requires. It is an analgesic and reduces nerve pain. The analgesic mechanism can affect the central nervous system; pain reduction may occur in this manner. Muira puama is a neuroprotectant and extends the life of your brain cells. It can enhance memory. The memory enhancement may be impressive for those with stress. Muira puama can treat depression, stress, anxiety, tics, neurasthenia, and Alzheimer's disease. This herb is as strong as almost any drug. You can try this on nerve problems associated with benign tumors. Keep your health care professional aware of all your supplements. Do not take this herb without supervision.

Siberian snow rose is very strong and has properties similar to those found in drugs. This herb may interact with blood-thinning agents and should not be taken by those on blood thinners without an Orthomolecular Medicine doctor's care and supervision. Another great herb to treat depression is used in combination with kefir yogurt and special mineral water. It is also a secret Russian anti-aging product. People from the Republic of Georgia drink Alpine tea on a daily basis with another product of kefir yogurt that has over ten probiotics.

Alpine tea is made with Siberian snow rose and water. The water in the Republic of Georgia is glacial water, with many glacial minerals. The anti-aging protocol of the Republic of Georgia consists of kefir yogurt, Alpine tea, glacial water, local wine, and honey. This protocol is very rich in flavonoids. The former Soviet Union has many herbal products that have been used as anti-aging tools by the wealthy for centuries. This nutritional anti-aging drink suggestion focuses on key minerals that help prevent and treat depression.

The Siberian snow rose and Alpine tea are used in hospitals in Asia to treat blood pressure problems, dementia, depression, neurosis, psychoses, memory, cognitive difficulties, and concentration problems. This herbal plant has antibiotic properties. It can slightly reduce fat storage, accelerate metabolism, and increase sweating. It can also lower blood pressure and is an important antioxidant. It increases blood circulation and passes through the blood-brain barrier. It helps stabilize brain activity and reduces capillary bleeding in the brain. It is unusual to increase brain circulation while reducing the likelihood of capillary bleeding in the brain.

The Siberian snow rose is unusual in that most herbal products that increase metabolism are not antioxidants. Many products that increase metabolism accelerate cellular aging and increase oxidation. It is interesting to note that the herb is not easily found around the world. It is not understood if this herb would work as well on people with different genotypes from other areas. People of Russian and Japanese descent should have great success with this product. It is important to use new products under the care and supervision of your health care professional. Quantum Brain Healing shares enthusiasm for the spectacular anti-aging and brain healing properties of Alpine tea.

Lemon balm treats primary brain disease or secondary brain symptoms from diseases targeting other body organs-diabetes, herpes, and cardiac diseases target specific organs but often have serious symptoms that coexist in the brain and remain undiagnosed. Depression is often a secondary disease that follows major diseases. Lemon balm is a great herb for its strong medical properties and mildness. Lemon balm can be grown in your garden and made as a tea. Quantum Brain Healing uses this herb as an antiviral and antibiotic agent. It can act as an antidepressant for mild depression.

Lemon balm is a sedative and antioxidant. It can be used to treat stress and anxiety. Its sedative effect can benefit nervous exhaustion. This herb acts on the brain in many ways to reduce signs of aging. Aging of the brain may be accelerated by bacterial and viral infections that go undiagnosed and untreated. Any herb that has antibiotic and antiviral actions may be taken on a regular basis to prevent this type of occurrence.

Saffron is used in Ayurvedic medicine as a stimulant and antioxidant. It inhibits platelet aggregation and helps prevent arteriosclerosis. It crosses the blood-brain barrier and increases circulation. Saffron prevents cancer, as well as preventing and slowing tumor formation. Saffron prevents mutation in DNA. This herb is a neuroprotectant.

Saffron can help treat headaches and depression that arise from insufficient blood circulation in the brain. These type of headaches and depression also may benefit from yoga and mild exercise. Saffron is useful in helping with alcoholism, but the addition of several amino acids is necessary as well. Milk thistle could also be included in the protocol for alcohol withdrawal, and two additional herbs chosen by your physician would be replaced as the patient progresses through the treatment.

The European herb piracetam changes the function of the right temporal lobe to increase brain circulation, increase cholinergic receptors in the brain, enhance memory, and act as a neuroprotectant. Piracetam may be used in treating many brain diseases, including amnesia, anxiety, depression, stroke, dyslexia, senility, Alzheimer's, and post-stroke aphasia. These brain diseases require other therapies along with piracetam for the best outcome.

Quantum Brain Healing uses vitamins, minerals, amino acids, nutritional supplements, and herbs in high doses to treat and heal brain disease. These supplements may be combined with other therapies. There may a focus on removing the toxins before adding the supplements.

Chinese club moss can increase energy levels, strengthen the immune system, increase alertness, improve learning, increase memory, impact neurotransmitter levels, and improve nerve function by strengthening and lengthening the nerve impulse. It can act as a brain enhancer.

Chinese club moss has treated many diseases, including Alzheimer's, myasthenia gravis, Parkinson's disease, memory loss, dementia, and cognitive impairment. Chinese club moss may be useful in reducing symptoms of Huntington's disease, multiple sclerosis, and spastic symptoms of undiagnosed diseases.

Chinese club moss must be combined with a proper diet and large quantities of many vitamins and minerals. Depression requires higher than the normally recommended daily levels of vitamins allowance normally required to improve health. Very large doses of many vitamins are needed for medicine or herbal products to achieve the best outcome. It is likely that once the body has a major disease, the level of vitamins and minerals needed for basic metabolism is increased. A major detoxification should be implemented early for those with depression, bipolar, multiple sclerosis, Huntington's, and Parkinson's diseases. Research is very inconclusive, but many theories suggest that toxic pesticides and chemicals are at the root of diseases and conditions like Alzheimer's, cognitive impairment, early dementia, and unexplained memory loss.

Milk thistle offers immune system enhancement and anti-inflammatory action. It is an antioxidant. This product can extend life and contribute to a healthier old age. Quantum Brain Healing uses this herb to treat addiction withdrawal, eating disorders, anxiety, and depression. Eating disorders may be a result of an impaired liver function, where the liver and gallbladder are over active. A well-functioning liver improves the outcome for many brain diseases. A healthy liver may result in less brain plaque or amyloid protein deposits in the brain.

A healthy liver is key to good health because this organ detoxifies the many chemicals and toxins that we are constantly exposed to and consume on a daily basis. Many times the liver is actually damaged by some of the more aggressive and toxic medicines. Impaired liver function is associated with depression in Chinese medicine. Poor liver function may be a result of liver enzyme problems or an overload of drug residue. Fatty livers can be treated successfully with amino acid therapy.

Milk thistle is a beneficial herb for most people and helps reduce toxins from the liver. Take this herb for seven to twelve weeks, and focus on improving liver function to heal depression. Spanish black radish supplements produced by Enzymatic Therapy are very good for improving liver health. Organic alfalfa, alpha lipoic acid, pectin, organic wheatgrass, and garlic supplements are very good detoxification agents for liver health. Fasting with juice or pure water can reduce toxins for the young and healthy; fasting is not recommended for those with serious brain diseases. Bikram yoga, or "hot yoga," will reduce toxins from your body. You must be sure to drink large quantities of pure water during any detoxification. You can remove years of damage to your liver with a carefully monitored detoxification. Improving your liver could also prevent eyesight problems and allow your eyes to focus better at night.

Acupuncture

Laser acupuncture is great for helping treat depression. A laser research study conducted with the Macquarie Center for Cognitive Sciences of New South Wales, Australia, found that laser stimulation on four acupuncture points used in Traditional Chinese Medicine stimulated the frontal-limber-striatal brain regions, with the pattern of brain activity varying with each different point. Brain areas with significantly increased activation included the limbic cortex and the frontal lobe. This action was demonstrated to be faster and more widespread than previously was understood. The limbic and frontal lobes are involved in anxiety, depression, and stress disorders.

Several studies have shown that laser acupuncture can benefit depression, memory loss, chronic fatigue, and cognitive disorders. Laser acupuncture and laser therapy are not for everyone; it is a therapy that is not widely available. Some doctors and acupuncturists use lasers that are inadequate and not strong enough to fully activate the body. There are also people using LED equipment and presenting this as laser therapy. The current LED is inadequate to cure depression.

There are many ways that laser therapy helps the brain. Bone health, autism, depression, stress, and sleep disorders involved with light activation may be benefit from laser therapy, including insomnia and hormone regulation. Laser therapy is the use of a beam of light to stimulate an area of the body or head. Laser therapy results in skin and surface activation, which occurs along with muscles and tendons. The stimulation of neurotransmitter production is also an important effect. Science has not fully explored the full range of health care benefits from laser therapy, so we do not know how long the effects will last for a given person.

Emotional Freedom Technique (EFT)

Emotional Freedom Technique, or EFT, is a therapy that excels at treating pain or symptoms related to emotional thoughts, feelings, trauma, or post-traumatic stress disorder (PTSD). Depression can be improved with EFT. This is a fairly inexpensive therapy that can be done with the help of a professional and reinforced by oneself at home. This therapy should be initially performed by an acupuncturist, chiropractor, Orthomolecular Medicine doctor, osteopath, or alternative medicine doctor.

EFT is a relatively new therapy that can benefit many people with disease and emotional trauma. It could alter the electro-magnetic field of the patient. This therapy, however, has not been extensively studied or published, and there are not adequate double-blind studies on this therapy in America.

EFT uses fingers to perform a tapping motion on acupuncture points along energy meridians established in Traditional Chinese Medicine. This is known as EFT tapping. This process is easy to perform on your own at home after a medical professional shows you the correct way to do the therapy. The points that are tapped on must be exactly correct in location. There may be additional points added to your treatment, depending upon your specific injury, disease, or level of emotional distress. This technique usually must be done more than once in order for it to succeed. Positive and negative affirmations are stated out loud while the tapping is done.

This therapy can alter your thoughts and feelings. Many diseases can improve or heal when the person changes his belief or thoughts concerning an illness or symptom. Many times, a patient's getting better can be as simple as getting someone to believe he can improve and helping him visualize this change in his life. Tapping may have this ability, along with moving the blocked energy along Chinese energy meridians. There are several energy meridians in the body, and they correspond to specific organs.

When the body's energy gets blocked or stuck in a specific organ, like the heart or small intestine, it may impact several organs and energy throughout the entire body. Chinese medicine believes that each energy meridian and organ is connected to emotions, directly or indirectly. As energetic blockages are removed and the energy flows freely, the person will improve and any emotionally caused problems can heal. It is possible for a person to get well in a single treatment, but many people will require several sessions. EFT will not replace hard work in overcoming addictions, but it will help in treating addictions and eating disorders. It can be used for healing depression, stress, anxiety, sleep disorders, migraines, seizures, and tics.

rTMS

Repetitive transcranial magnetic stimulation (rTMS) is a noninvasive method for applying electromagnetic fields to the brain. Application is through a medical device with a low 0.9 hertz frequency stimulation. It requires more than one session. One of the side effects is a tendency to underestimate time. Another side effect may be a slight headache. It is contraindicated in epilepsy and multiple sclerosis.

Single sessions of rTMS placed over the temporal or temporoparietal cortex can cure a very short-term problem with tinnitus (ringing in your ears). Repeated sessions of rTMS may successfully treat tinnitus, but the treatment is not known to cure tinnitus. The results are variable. It may have more success for those whose problem is due to long-term effects of drug addiction. This treatment may also be useful for some forms of hearing loss that are not noise-induced. Hearing loss from medications and diseases may find some help with rTMS.

This treatment affects the auditory cortex and may help other problems associated with the auditory cortex, including depression, memory problems in the motor cortex, and flashbacks. The therapy was used on a patient with major depression, five times per week, and it was successful. It is very hard to treat major depression, and this may turn out to be one of the best options. This treatment is noninvasive and causes no pain. The treatment may have results that extend beyond the motor cortex area of the brain.

Bio-Mat

The Bio-Mat is a device that uses far infrared and amethyst crystals. The patient lies on the mat for twenty or thirty minutes and listens through earphones to sounds and instructions. It seems like a meditation session, and it relaxes your body as the infrared speeds the elimination of toxins. It also ionizes your body with negative ions, which improves your body's ability to heal. This should normally be used about twice a week on the depression patient. The Bio-Mat, however, is not inexpensive—it can cost upwards of $2,500, depending on the size you choose—but it is a unique device. It is a patented device, and there is one manufacturer.

Hemi-Sync and Metatones

Quantum Brain Healing uses many therapies to help the brain recover, along with Orthomolecular Medicine. One of the most innovative types of biofeedback is Hemi-Sync, created by Dr. Robert Monroe. It is a space-age concept of entraining the brain waves into the desired state to heal a specific disease. Your brain waves may become irregular when you develop certain brain conditions. Entraining is the concept of coaxing your brain waves into the pattern being played into your ears with Hemi-Sync. You can find the Hemi-Sync CD systems online at reasonable prices. The CD's may be played in a portable CD player with headphones. The sound helps balance or heal your brain.

Dr. Monroe developed a type of brain biofeedback that synchronized brain waves and altered the brain-wave activity and balance between the left and right hemispheres to increase peak performance level. In order to reduce mental impairment of almost any type, imbalances in the brain waves need correction, and this can be achieved through extended exposure to the proper frequencies with a binaural beat. Binaural beats occur when different frequencies are delivered to the right and left hemispheres of the brain simultaneously.

Neurophysiologist are researching binaural beats to determine their impact on hearing. Binaural beats are also studied for their ability to entrain brain waves and their use for relaxation and health benefits. This is based upon the concept that brain disabilities and impairments are due to emotionally altered vibrations from your mind. These alter the auric energy field of your brain in a negative way to change the type of brain wave or make the pattern of any type of brain wave irregular.

Dr. Monroe's research has been taken to the next level in the research as Metatones. Metatones can be used to treat depression, anxiety, epilepsy, autism, addiction, learning disabilities, dementia, ADD, insomnia, PTSD, Alzheimer's, dyslexia, ADHD, closed head injury, and moderate eating disorders. This therapy is worth trying for people with brain conditions that do not respond to typical therapy and is a drug-free option. If more than one family member has an addiction disorder or learning disability, the product can be used for each of them. This is not a suitable therapy, however, for people with hearing problems.

Music Therapy

Quantum Brain Healing relies on a large group of supplements, including amino acids, vitamins, minerals, and herbs. These are integrated into an overall program that includes detoxification of chemicals, toxins, and pesticides. After the toxins are removed, a healthy diet of organic vegetables and fruits will help people regain health quickly. Food-based multivitamins are included for most people.

For some people, this is not enough, and adjunct therapies en masse will be used for very hard cases. Metatones is auditory vibrational energy therapy that addresses problems of ADD, ADHD, epilepsy, learning disabilities, autism, addiction, depression, dyslexia, head trauma, insomnia, PTSD, stroke, MS, and Alzheimer's. The brain can be balanced with amino acids to assist with neurotransmitter rebalancing, and auditory therapy can also indirectly affect neurotransmitter levels.

Music therapy, Acutonics (sound healing education), singing, and Tibetan singing bowls are simpler versions of the concept of using music or sound vibrations to heal. The Hemi-Sync Method is a more sophisticated version of vibrational sound therapy developed by Dr. Robert Monroe. The brain can be balanced by auditory therapy. The sounds are played on a CD and listened to with headphones. The brain-wave activity is altered by the sound vibration as it is heard. There are several types of brain waves, and your brain may not experience proper brain-wave activity.

Research shows that Parkinson's and Alzheimer's brains have decidedly different brain waves than the normal brain. Hemi-Sync works to entrain the brain into the proper brain-wave activity for health. Vibrational energy healing is based on the tenet that disease stems from a lack of proper resonance. This is relatively inexpensive method—just the cost of the CDs—and you can play the CDs as many times as you need. Music therapy and sound therapy have had successful results.

Most forms of medicine believe that disease is rooted by a lack of balance. Health will return when the cell is put into vibrational balance. It seems that music therapy may be one more way in which to influence and change neurotransmitter levels. Classical music and baroque music are the best music for balancing the brain. Music therapy with a harp has been used to treat MS. Learning to play the piano or guitar can help balance the brain of a child with ADD or ADHD. Singing upbeat songs is a great way for a child to improve her depression. Stroke patients who are unable to speak may be able to hum along with music.

Medical devices that are understood to help treat depression include:

- ➢ Alpha-Stim 100, an electrical stimulation device that clips onto the earlobes
- ➢ Acupuncture electro-stimulation attaches electrical stimulation to acupuncture needles
- ➢ Electrical stimulation of the auricular acupuncture points with a hand held electrical stimulation device
- ➢ Transcranial magnetic stimulation
- ➢ Medical-grade laser therapy on auricular acupuncture points

➢ Surgical implantation of electrical electrodes under the skin

➢ Magnetic stimulation of auricular points with small retention magnets

Other therapies that have helped depression include biofeedback, NAET, EFT, BEST, laser therapy, detoxification, and cranial sacral therapy.

DYSLEXIA

Dyslexia is a brain malfunction in the left parietal lobe, left temporal lobe, and the Wernicke's area. The brain problems stem from language-processing areas in the left hemisphere of the brain. Dyslexia is a learning disability that affects reading, spelling, and math. Dyslexia creates a situation where a person with average or above average intelligence performs at lower levels.

People with dyslexia are often gifted in areas controlled by the right hemisphere of the brain, which includes artistic skill, musical ability, mechanical ability, three-dimensional spatial skills, intuition, creativity, global thinking, curiosity, athletic ability, and drive. People with dyslexia frequently are outstanding in music, scientific research, psychology, architecture, interior or exterior design, teaching, marketing and sales, culinary arts, woodworking, carpentry, performing arts, athletics, engineering, computers, electronics, mechanics, graphic arts, and photography.

Alternative medicine treatments for aphasia, which is often associated with stroke, will often improve and achieve lasting recoveries for some dyslexic patients. Please review those listed therapies shown in the chapter on stroke for additional externally applied and non-dietary treatment options.

Researchers at Maastricht University in the Netherlands have discovered that dyslexic people exhibit less neural activity with less activation of the superior temporal cortex region of the temporal lobe of the brain. Research also shows that families with autism often have depression and/or dyslexia. Prognosis for dyslexia improves when there is a second language learned. Enroll the child in a second and third language class, and he or she will succeed and recover.

Dyslexia has little to do with intelligence. Albert Einstein and Leonardo da Vinci both had dyslexia. It often runs in families and is genetic in nature. The dyslexic may have poor nonverbal skills and may be slow to learn to read. It affects short-term verbal memory, motor skills, spelling ability, and written language. There is uneven or unpredictable performance from day to day. The dyslexic person often confuses right and left and up and down. This person has problems with numbers and numerical order. The child's homework may be very messy and have crossed-out areas or writing on top of other writing. Dyslexia creates difficulty with following directions of instructions in a classroom setting. The dyslexic person may fail to recognize words or include extra words into his speech. This person requires higher concentration levels and energy in order to learn and becomes more easily exhausted from learning than the average student.

It is extremely important to increase the self-esteem of children with dyslexia. Reading problems can lead to being perceived as less intelligent. It is important to increase the nonverbal skills of these children and increase their group skills. Developing areas of skill that are not related to the classroom can increase self-esteem. Hobbies, sports, music, and games will all develop the brain and improve self-esteem. People always perform better in a classroom when they have high self-esteem. Low self-esteem leads people to feel as though there is no point in trying.

Dyslexia is lifelong and varies in severity. It can accompany ADD, ADHD, autism, and Asperger's syndrome. The pharmaceutical drugs Ritalin or Adderall can help the most severe of cases if used on a short-term basis during crisis periods. It is not a solution, however, and should not be used longer than two weeks. The prognosis for dyslexia is good if diagnosed early and treated. The herbal alternative to using Ritalin or Adderall as a stimulant is a combination of choline, lemon balm, guarana, and piracetam. This combination can be used in combination with the Alpha-Stim 100 to stimulate the Wernicke's area of the brain. Attach the ear clips to the child about two to three times per week for twenty minutes, and set the device at a low level. Take the combination of herbals about forty minutes to an hour prior to using the device. The combination should be taken once a day for three to six months to determine the success of this treatment protocol.

Ginkgo biloba is also a stimulating brain herb that crosses the blood-brain barrier and stimulates the temporal lobe. The dyslexic child should be closely monitored by a naturopath, doctor, or orthomolecular physician during the year to two years of using the Alpha-Stim 100 and herb combination treatment—it usually requires at least this long to significantly improve the patient. Reading programs can be added to further develop the brain. The dyslexic child will have to work harder for years to reach his or her potential. He or she can become a top-level student, however, and make it through medical school or a PhD program.

Diet is important with any learning disability. There are several dietary suggestions; if one does not help, try another. Avoiding additives and toxins is very important. Check for nutritional deficiencies through diagnostic testing. Correcting nutritional deficiencies often has a large impact on brain function and learning. Diagnostic testing for heavy metals must be done if there is a chance of exposure. Detoxification of heavy metals includes proper diet, herbs, nutritional supplements, far infrared sauna, and foot ionizing detoxification. A weight-loss program is needed if the patient is overweight and toxins of all types, including heavy metals, are stored in fat cells.

Many environmental allergies can make existing learning disabilities worse. Check your house for mold, pesticides, and heavy metals. NAET is a great therapy to eliminate allergies.

There are many alternative treatments for dyslexia, and some are more effective than others. I would start with dietary changes, nutritional supplements, auricular acupuncture, herbs, and the Tomatis method (defined as "a pedagogy of listening"). Dietary and nutritional changes are synergistic with the other treatments. Monitor the amount of time the child spends in front of the computer and television to avoid excess stimulation. Spend time outdoors when possible.

Alternative treatments that can help dyslexia include:

- Neurofeedback
- Auricular therapy
- Scalp acupuncture
- Chinese herbal formula
- NAET
- Music therapy
- Sound therapy
- Hemi-Sync by the Monroe Institute
- Quantum healing
- Radionics
- BEST
- Craniosacral therapy
- Listening therapy
- Vibrational medicine
- Homeopathy

Hemi-Sync involves binaural beating, a sensory-information stimulus, and changes the information sent to the reticular-thalamic activating system, which improves attention, focus, and level of awareness. Hemi-Sync signals contribute to a greater balance of activity of the right and left hemispheres and cortical and subcortical areas of the brain. Hemi-Sync is used to improve dyslexia, Asperger's, Down's syndrome, autism, learning disabilities, developmentally disabled, ADHD, OCD, brain trauma, bipolar disorder, cerebral palsy, seizure disorders, and to improve cognitive function in children with borderline IQ. Children who are deaf, who have a unilateral hearing loss, or who have an absence of a brain structure such as the corpus callosum improve with Hemi-Sync. This also would be a good therapy for most people after brain surgery to speed their recovery and help regain maximum brain function.

Dietary suggestions include:

- Eliminate sugar, refined foods, carbonated beverages, alcohol
- Focus on organic food, when available
- Gluten-free diet
- Casein-free diet (no milk products)
- Additive-free diet
- Elimination diet
- Caffeine-free diet
- Increase green vegetables
- Increase dietary fiber

Nutritional supplements that can help dyslexia include:

- Omega-3 fatty acids
- Omega-6 fatty acids
- Super blue-green algae
- Pycnogenol
- DHEA
- PS (phosphatidylserine)
- Choline
- Lecithin
- DMAE
- L-carnitine
- Tyrosine
- Probiotics
- Alpha lipoic acid

Quantum Brain Healing treats dyslexia with lithium orotate, the trace mineral salt found in RNA and DNA, which is used for repairing damaged nerves. Lithium orotate is one of several trace mineral salts that is commonly used in naturopathic medicine. It can travel inside the brain to stabilize many of the chemical activities of the neurons and protects brain cells in the hippocampus, striatum, and frontal cortex of the brain. It helps stimulate the growth of new neurons.

Another use of lithium orotate is for stress-induced memory loss. It is also good for violent outbursts. It can stabilize the brain during periods of extremely irregular brain-wave activity. Lithium orotate increases neural plasticity, which is important for preserving or increasing intelligence. Children with dyslexia should try this option for no more than five days. If treat results are achieved, lithium orotate can be seriously monitored and used. Otherwise, discontinue use immediately.

Quantum Brain Healing uses this trace mineral salt to treat alcoholism. Adults with dyslexia and alcoholism may be helped with this supplement. These diseases may benefit from its ability to stabilize neurons, grown new neurons, and add to neural plasticity. Additional support should be added for alcohol withdrawal if this is a problem.

Herbs

> Piracetam (enhances reading ability in dyslexia)

> Lemon balm

> Guarana

> Ginkgo biloba

> Panax ginseng

> Gotu kola

> Catuaba

> Eleutherococcus senticosus

> Fo-Ti (root)

> Da zao

> Organic decaffeinated green tea

> Skullcap

> Butcher's broom

> Valerian (to increase concentration, reasoning skills, and motor coordination)

Catuaba is a South American herb that has many medicinal properties, including the ability to act as an antibiotic and antiviral. It also is an adaptogen and analgesic and can sedate or stimulate the brain and central nervous system as needed. Catuaba can treat dyslexia. Use this herb on a daily basis at night, forty-four minutes before bed.

Catuaba should not be considered a sole treatment; it should be combined with nutritional supplements, including amino acids. 5-HTP, GABA, or SAM-e can contribute to faster balancing of neurotransmitters. Catuaba is a primary herb, along with valerian, lemon balm, ginkgo biloba, and vinpocetine, for treating dyslexia. A liver detoxification and heavy-metals detoxification prior to the use of catuaba usually improves or hastens its success. Quantum Brain Healing relies on the use of therapeutic minerals and vitamins to rebalance the body. The key factor of catuaba is that it is an adaptogen.

Lemon balm is another primary herb. This herb will help approximately 35-45 percent of those with dyslexia. It can be used by children ages nine and older. Lemon balm inhibits the production of the thyroid hormone and could help treat Hashimoto's disease in its early phase. It can also treat hyperthyroid or Graves' disease. Do not take this herb if you have hypothyroid disease or take thyroid medicine. Lemon balm acts on the hippocampus area of the brain and functions as an antispasmodic. Lemon balm is a sedative, antibiotic, antiviral, and antioxidant and is an acetylcholinesterase inhibitor. This herb acts on the brain in many ways to reduce signs of aging. Aging of the brain may be accelerated by bacterial and viral infections.

A clinical trial was recently conducted on fifteen dyslexic children, aged five to thirteen, with ginkgo biloba. The results are good and suggest that an extract of ginkgo biloba (EGb 761) at doses up to 80 mg/day may lessen the learning difficulty associated with dyslexia. The 80 mg was taken in the morning. The children were not taking psychotropic medication during the trial. There is a need for a double-blind trial. The main side effect in the clinical trial reported was a brief headache was reported by two of the children.

Auricular Therapy

Auricular therapy acupuncture of the ear—is a way to treat the entire body with acupuncture points located on the ear. This alternative medicine therapy mobilizes endorphins and enkephalin opioid peptides, increases serotonin and dopamine neurotransmitters, and increases levels of substance P and cholecystokinin (CCK). Auricular acupuncture helps the body in balancing levels of stress and sex hormones. It reduces cortisol, glucose levels, and the body's overall inflammation level. Auricular therapy modulates neurotransmitters and is very helpful in dealing with substance abuse recovery and mood disorders. Try auricular therapy along with scalp and body acupuncture for good results.

Auricular therapy can include needles, electrical stimulation, laser therapy, or electro-acupuncture. Auricular acupuncture is one therapy that can be used to treat dyslexia. Quantum Brain Healing suggests retention needles in the ears for two to four hours per treatment. Electro-acupuncture is a great tool; taking supplements and herbal formulas one hour before acupuncture treatments may speed progress. Dyslexia can be reduced within fifteen minutes of application of auricular therapy to certain auricular acupuncture points by applying electrical stimulation to the ear.

The auricular acupuncture points for treating dyslexia include:

- Occiput
- Shen men
- Subcortex
- Brain
- Neurasthenia
- Sympathetic

Chinese diagnosis: Dyslexia may be caused by essence deficiency, blood deficiency, blood stagnation, and other syndromes.

Acupuncture Points

Yong Quan (KI-1), Shen Men (HT-7), Xin Shu (BL-15), Bai Hui (GV-20), and Lie Que (LU-7). Two adjunctive points were mentioned at least three times: Zu San Li (ST-36) and Hou Xi (SI-3).

Chinese Herbal Formula

- Jie Yu Dan or aphasia pill
- Relaxing speech pill

These Chinese Patent formulas are available through a Chinese herbalist or an acupuncture physician. Traditional Chinese Medicine (TCM) actions for these formulas indicate that they calm wind, transform phlegm, open the orifices, and increase circulation in the channels. Western medical indications for these TCM formulas include dyslexia, aphasia, sequelae of cerebrovascular accident, stuttering, paralysis of the limbs, and weakness of the limbs.

Quantum Brain Healing likes using TCM patent formulas but wants the general public to understand that these should be prescribed by an acupuncturist, naturopath, or herbalist. The use of formulas for children should be very carefully monitored.

NeuroCare NC10004PXP

This medical device is based on low amperage technology and should never be confused with other neurofeedback devices or brain-stimulating devices. It can be used to treat many brain illnesses, including depression, insomnia, anxiety, and addictions. Its other medical uses include diabetic wound care, muscle atrophy, paralysis from trauma, post-surgical recovery, prevention of deep vein thrombosis, and increasing local circulation.

The treatment of dyslexia requires a commitment to several treatments per week for one to years and monthly sessions lasting forty minutes for seven years. It is possible to notice improvement after fourteen sessions. The sessions should take approximately twelve to twenty minutes, three times per week for the first month. The treatments should last about sixteen to twenty-four minutes per session during the second month. The treatments during the third month should last twenty-one to twenty-nine minutes. The treatments during the fourth month should take twenty-seven to thirty-five minutes per session. If there are any negative reactions or serious pain, discontinue the session. The following session should go back to the previous level without problems.

NeuroCare NC10004PXP equipment is expensive, and your doctor may require you to pay a deposit up front and commit to a number of sessions if he orders the equipment specifically to treat you.

Ondamed

Ondamed is a small medical device that could be considered a combination of neurofeedback for the emotions and an electromagnetic stimulus to energize electron flow and oscillate cells in a range of .1 to 32,000 Hz. It is believed to help manage emotional trauma and reduce inflammation and stress. It enhances lymphatic flow, improves metabolism, and affects the nervous system. Dyslexia can cause emotional trauma - it can be very traumatic for a child or teenager to have poor performance in school.

Ondamed may treat hidden emotions stored on a cellular level that negatively affect the immune system. This treatment may require several sessions before there is noticeable improvement. You should expect to commit to at least thirty to forty treatments for dyslexia. Dyslexic teens with an addiction may require a sessions lasting about seven minutes longer and require more treatments than those with simple dyslexia. Teenagers with dyslexia have higher than average experimentation rates with tobacco and recreational drugs. These teenagers are more likely to become addicts and suffer from anxiety.

Auditory Integration Training (AIT)

Distortions in hearing or auditory processing in the brain contribute to behavioral or learning disorders such as autism spectrum disorder. Auditory integration training (AIT) is a controversial therapy, but it may be useful in treating dyslexia, autism spectrum disorder, anxiety, depression, ADD, ADHD, central auditory processing disorders (CAPD), speech disorders, sensory disorders, and pervasive developmental disorder (PDD). This therapy will not work for many people, but where hearing problems have the largest impact on the patient, it could be extremely useful. An example of this type of problem is a difference in hearing ability between the left and right ears. This will result in a processing challenge in the brain. Disorganized messages may be transmitted to the CNS as a result.

AIT may help in correcting or improving auditory processing problems that may occur if the auditory messages received by the brain are distorted. It is also used for hypersensitivity to sound. AIT involves listening to vocal music through headphones connected to a device that electronically transforms the sounds. These sessions require thirty minutes, typically twice a day for ten consecutive days. Before receiving the AIT, the individual is given an audiogram to determine the hearing ability for various sound frequencies. After this, the individual listens to music through a special machine through the earphones. Although no scientific research exists to support this intervention, some parents feel it has made significant changes for their child. Others have noted few if any differences after the therapy. Supposedly, AIT reduces hearing hypersensitivity for some people, as well as providing intense stimulation for the brain.

Alpha-Stim 100

This small medical device is prescribed by doctors and acupuncturists and is slightly larger than a deck of cards. It has wires that attach to ear clips. Each ear clip has a small pad where several drops of a liquid are placed before the clips are attached to your ear lobes. The time and frequency are set at your prescribed levels. The device operates with a D battery. This device may be worn several times per week. It treats many brain illnesses. There has not been a clinical trial for this use; however, the machine has been found to be useful cases with some similar symptoms. It require a medium frequency setting and short amount of time. This should be tried about fifteen sessions prior to calling its success. If you experience pain, dial back the frequency until the pain subsides and continue wearing the device. Inform your doctor immediately, as the Alpha-Stim 100 has not been tested for this use.

It is useful in at altering neurotransmitter levels and has been used on children. It may take approximately at least one year of treatments before the reading improvements and brain function improvement are permanent. The sessions should be nine to twelve minutes for four or five days per week. The setting on the machine can be gradually increased. There is research to document its ability to improve concentration, memory, and learning skills.

EnerMed

The EnerMed is a non-invasive, battery-operated, electromagnetic device, about the size of a large watch. The EnerMed emits a weak, pulsed electromagnetic wave that is specific for each patient. It has been used in clinical trials to treat and improve multiple sclerosis and migraines.

The brain has a wide range of electromagnetic frequencies. Many brains have irregular brain-wave activity, and the neurons fire irregularly or less often than they should. These irregular brain waves can be corrected in several ways such as neurofeedback or binaural stimulation. The EnerMed device can produce electromagnetic stimulation at a specific frequency to repair, treat, or heal a diseased brain. The frequency that is needed depends on the brain disorder. People suffering from depression, anxiety, Alzheimer's, migraines, ADHD, dyslexia, and multiple sclerosis usually have irregular brain frequencies.

When the brain wave and frequencies are balanced, many neurological symptoms improve. The EnerMed device is used to stimulate these specific frequencies and restore the body's natural balance. Your EnerMed device will generate pulsed electromagnetic stimulation at these frequencies to restore homeostasis to your neuromodulatory systems. It is set specifically for your set of symptoms and illness. It has been called a "pacemaker for the brain." This device has not been specifically tested for dyslexia. It may be capable of seriously improving approximately one-half of people with dyslexia who are diagnosed and treated early.

Music Therapy

Music or sound therapy can be used to treat dyslexia on the physical, emotional, and cognitive levels of the disease. Music or sound therapy is the application of sound waves from a voice, tuning fork, harp, computer, or alternative electronic device to rebalance or increase a person's vibrations. Drumming and chanting are forms of Native American music therapy, which are successfully used to correct health problems.

Music works to heal the patient and rebalance his energy through the energetic principles of resonance and entrainment. Music affects the synchronization between the right and left hemispheres of the brain and the electrical voltage produced in the brain. Music can directly affect the brain and endocrine system, altering neurotransmitters and hormones. Music can change the production of dopamine and serotonin, which are involved in pleasure, reward, arousal, motivation, and memory. It can stimulate or sedate the patient. Classical music can reduce cortisol, a stress-related hormone. Listening to classical music may benefit any person with diabetes or metabolic disorder, influencing cortisol's effect on insulin. Listening to Mozart has reduced epileptic seizures by 65 percent. Research has showed that patients listening to music several hours a day for three months improved their verbal memory by 60 percent and improved their ability to control and perform mental operations.

The Tomatis Method (Listening Therapy)

Sound-wave therapy was developed in Europe in the 1950s when Dr. Peter Manners developed a machine to heal with vibrations. The machine was placed on the afflicted area and a frequency was matched vibration of the cells of a healthy body. After the Tomatis treatment with vibrations, the afflicted area resonated with a higher frequency.

Dr. Manners developed a computerized system with about eight hundred frequencies used to treat a range of conditions. Other therapies that pursue this concept are bio-resonance and vibrational therapy. Sound-wave therapy is used to treat a wide range of diseases.

Dr. Alfred Tomatis and Dr. Guy Berard took this technology and incorporated it into auditory integration training, where the patient listens to sounds through headphones. Listening therapy is the method developed by Dr. Tomatis (the Tomatis method) to treat conditions including dyslexia, learning disabilities, ADHD, Down's syndrome, autism, depression, anxiety, behavioral problems, and chronic fatigue in both children and adults.

Interactive Metronome Therapy

Interactive metronome (IM) therapy was developed to improve learning and developmental disorders in children. It is also effective for adults in brain rehabilitation. IM is a neuromotor assessment and treatment tool used in therapy to improve the neurological processes of motor planning and sequencing. IM improves motor planning and sequencing by using neurosensory and neuromotor exercises to increase brain plasticity.

The human brain's efficiency and performance depend on the seamless transition of neuron network signals from one area of the brain to another. The research of Neal Alpiner, MD, suggests that IM works by augmenting internal processing speed within the neuroaxis. The brain is affected in the cerebellum, prefrontal cortex, cingulate gyrus, and basal ganglia. This area is responsible for sustained attention, language formulation, motor coordination, and balance.

The IM program provides a structured, goal-oriented process that challenges the patient to synchronize a range of hand and foot exercises to a precise computer-generated reference tone heard through headphones. IM requires a series of twelve to fifteen sessions. It works through listening to a rhythmic sound through stereo headphones and responding by tapping or clapping and attempting to match the beat. A patented auditory-visual guidance system provides immediate feedback measured in milliseconds, and a score is provided.

IM trains the brain to learn rhythm and timing. As timing improves, so do motor control, coordination, focus, concentration, language processing, aggression, impulsiveness, endurance, strength, filtering out distractions, attention span, self-control, school performance, and social performance. IM has been used to treat dyslexia, sensory integration disorder, ADHD, traumatic brain injury (TBI), cerebral vascular accident (CVA), autism spectrum disorder, cerebral palsy, non-verbal learning disorder, Asperger's syndrome, delayed speech development, Parkinson's disease, and balance problems.

Irlen Syndrome Treatment with Colored Lenses

Irlen syndrome—a visual perceptual problem in which people see distortion on a page of numbers, words, or musical notes—may be a type of dyslexia. Irlen syndrome affects the individual's reading, spelling, math, problem solving, copying skills, music reading, driving, sports performance, and working on a computer. Wireless internet and fluorescent lights make this problem worse.

Those afflicted with Irlen syndrome constantly adapt to the distortions their brain creates when viewing a printed page. They may be slow readers because of this or have low comprehension and reduced attention span. This also causes eye strain and fatigue. People with dyslexia or Irlen syndrome are often seen as underachievers with behavioral or attitude issues. American psychologist Helen Irlen first defined this problem and found a solution: specially formulated colored overlays or colored lenses that can be worn as glasses or even contact lenses. The Irlen Method improves the brain's ability to process visual information, which then improves concentration and reduces mistakes.

Reflexology

Reflexology promotes relaxation and reduces stress. It is based on the principle that the anatomy of the body is reflected in miniature reflex zones on the head, ears, hands, and feet. Dyslexia can be improved with reflexology on the face and the feet. The face treatment should occur before reflexology on the feet. The facial reflexologist should spend extra time around the ears and nose; the facial reflexology treatment should last at least nine minutes, and the remaining time should be spent on the feet.

Sessions typically last sixty minutes. Both feet are worked on, one at time, during the session. The reflexologist will gently massage the feet and apply pressure to the reflex points that correlate to your health problems. With dyslexia, pressure is applied to the reflex points that correlate to the brain, brain stem, heart, liver, and adrenal. Reflexology is similar to the concept of acupressure. Some reflexologists apply pressure with their fingers while others use small instruments.

People with foot problems, such as severe calluses or corns, should visit a podiatrist for treatment prior to a reflexology treatment. Dyslexia requires the manipulation of the feet to remove any tiny calcium crystals that accumulate in the nerve endings of the feet. Another way to reinforce this action on the feet is to purchase an infrared foot massager. Foot ionizing detoxification also may help remove excess calcium and ferrous iron buildup from the feet.

Reflexology restores the qi, or free flow of energy, from the feet to the corresponding organs. Pressure on the reflex points may trigger the release of hormones, including endorphins, chemicals in the brain that naturally block pain. Reflexology relaxes the face, improves circulation, and increases the rate at which detoxification occurs. Reflexology should be used in addition to other therapies.

rTMS

Repetitive transcranial magnetic stimulation (rTMS) is a noninvasive method for applying electromagnetic fields to the brain. Application is through a medical device with a low 0.9 hertz frequency stimulation. It requires more than one session to be effective. One of the side effects of rTMS is a tendency to underestimate time. Another side effect may be a slight headache. Use of rTMS is contraindicated for those with epilepsy and multiple sclerosis.

This therapy is not commonly used for dyslexia and has not been frequently used on children or teenagers, but it may be useful for older teenagers and young adults with significant dyslexia. Do not use rTMS for those with few symptoms. It would be very helpful if dyslexia patients were given detoxification for heavy metals and pesticides prior to administering the rTMS. Oral chelation with formulas available in health food stores and products like rutin, chorella, organic wheatgrass, organic barley capsules, cilantro, aloe, parsley, garlic, algae, grapefruit pectin, and alpha lipoic acid—will safely remove toxins over time. It will take approximately six to twelve months to remove most of the toxins found in a middle-aged adult. Saunas can accomplish this with about three to twelve sessions, lasting about thirty minutes each. The rTMS may be used approximately one month after aggressive oral chelation has started.

Single sessions of rTMS placed over the temporal or temporoparietal cortex may improve dyslexia. Use no more than three sessions of rTMS on those younger than nineteen. The results are variable. It may have more success for those with dyslexia who have abused drugs. This treatment affects the auditory cortex and may help other problems associated with the auditory cortex, including memory problems in the motor cortex, flashbacks, and depression. The therapy was used for major depression on a patient, five times per week, and was successful. This treatment is noninvasive and causes no pain. It may have results that extend beyond the motor cortex area of the brain.

Some studies indicate that rTMS increases brain plasticity and could have the ability to increase intelligence, given the optimal combination of brain nutrients and other alternative therapies. This treatment may be a way to enhance learning and increase memory. rTMS could be wonderful for those with memory and learning disabilities connected to head trauma, brain injuries, and memory loss due to cardiac problems from low oxygen levels in the brain. Take 400 - 700 mg of alpha lipoic acid approximately fifty-four minutes prior to treatment with rTMS.

Speed Learning

Dyslexia can be improved up to 300 percent, along with math scores, memory training, increased comprehension, concentration, vocabulary, and learning skills, with a program called Speed Learning. This would benefit any family with young children or older people re-entering college. With frequent daily sessions for three months to a year, this program can help improve dyslexia.

Speed Learning can more than double your ability to learn math, language, and memory skills. This technique has been changed since the early seventies and now includes rhythms and frequencies. The program is available online and can be shared by one than one child in a family. The information on the program and the summary of their experiments can be found in the book *Superlearning*. This previously expensive technology is now available on a CD for $19.95 plus tax and shipping at the website.

EPILEPSY

Quantum Brain Healing uses acupuncture for treating and healing epilepsy. Seizures are due to abnormal electrical activity. Seizure disorders differ from epilepsy and these seizures of unknown origin are often treated or cured far more easily than epilepsy. Seizures may occur due to allergies to food or medicine. Patients should be tested and treated for food allergies early in the process. Seizures may occur due to head trauma, epilepsy, or heavy-metals toxins. Seizures may also result from exposure to carbon monoxide or sarin gas. Sarin gas is a poison gas that was used in the subway in Japan to kill and harm many people in a terrorist act. Exposure to large quantities of chlorine gas can cause a seizure. When one understands the triggers for seizures, it can make the condition less traumatic.

Epileptic seizures may be triggered by vitamin and mineral deficiencies, food allergies, stress, environmental toxins and allergens, physical or emotional trauma, neurotoxins (such as aspartame), allergic reactions to pharmaceutical drugs, recreational drug abuse, stimulants, sleep deprivation, strobe light exposure, low blood sugar, extreme temperature exposure (either hot or cold), and dehydration. Many types of illness can produce seizures in a crisis stage. It is uncommon, but a diabetic patient whose glucose levels are extremely low or high may experience a seizure.

One-half of epileptic patients have abnormal carbohydrate metabolism, resulting in hypoglycemia. Low blood sugar can trigger a seizure or cause the person to faint. Eating can stave off a seizure if the epileptic person closely monitors symptoms of hypoglycemia. Epileptic patients have low levels of vitamin B1, vitamin B6, calcium, manganese, zinc, and magnesium; they are often deficient in L-cysteine.

Alcoholism is often prevalent in families of epilepsy patients. There is clear evidence that even one drink of alcohol can trigger an epileptic seizure for some people. Seizures may be due to an allergic reaction to alcohol by the epileptic person. There is also a high incidence of constipation for many people with epilepsy. Constipation allows toxins to build up in the colon, which may trigger epileptic seizures. A colon cleanse, enema, high-fiber diet, and fiber supplement can reduce the likelihood of this event.

The use of organic products and organic food is very important. Other areas of importance include minimizing toxic household cleaning items and improving air quality with an ionizing household air filter. Try to avoid commonly encountered pesticides, such as dieldrin, lindane, and the pyrethroids which interfere with the brain's electrical activity of the brain. Pesticides and other toxins can bind with benzodiazepine receptors and cause seizures or convulsions in some people. Energy disruption through exposure to excessive electromagnetic fields can cause seizures in susceptible people. Try to avoid areas where there are too many cell phone towers and wireless systems in one place.

Heavy-metals toxins such as lead, mercury, cadmium, titanium, and aluminum interfere with proper nerve function and can cause seizures or convulsions. Dental amalgam contains mercury, which crosses the blood-brain barrier. This alters brain activity and neurotransmitters levels. Research studies show that epilepsy can improve after removal of dental amalgam. Quantum Brain Healing goes into detail about which heavy metals cause specific problems associated with brain seizures.

Hormone Dysfunction

There is a correlation between menstruation and associated seizure patterns. Imbalances of estrogen and progesterone definitely have an impact in seizure activity in premenopausal women. A good way to understand this connection is to keep a diary of seizure activity and one's menstrual cycle. It is important to get baseline hormone tests results initially.

If there is an imbalance, one can supplement with herbs, such as vitex to increase progesterone levels, or red clover, which binds with estrogen receptor sites to manage hormone levels. This can also be accomplished with bio-identical hormones. Bio-identical hormones are taken on a long-term basis and can be fairly expensive. There are more affordable Chinese patent herbal formulas which can produce similar results. The bio-identical hormones may be easier on the stomach or more absorbable for some patients.

Acupuncture

There are indications that in order to achieve long-term relief, acupuncture treatment needs to be continued on a regular basis for a period of two years. Dietary changes and detoxification of heavy metals should occur shortly after diagnosis. Scalp, body, and auricular acupuncture are successful in treatment of epilepsy. Quantum Brain Healing often uses acupuncture points in treating epilepsy and the range of seizure symptoms. Additional therapies that may be considered are vagus nerve stimulation, acupuncture, scalp acupuncture, auricular acupuncture, and electro-acupuncture to treat brain inflammation.

Acupuncture may also function as a neuroprotectant for patients with epilepsy or seizure disorders. Chinese herbal formulas are a neuroprotectant, immune enhancer, anti-anxiety, and anti-inflammatory. Chinese medicine can treat many diseases successfully that remain unresolved with Western medicine. Seizures of unknown origin can be treated or cured with Traditional Chinese Medicine. Early diagnosis and treatment with acupuncture in children can produce remarkable results. Most of these types of seizures of unknown origin are treated with little success by allopathic medicine. Epilepsy is not cured overnight, and often herbal formulas are used on a long-term basis.

Medical researchers have showed that acupuncture produces autonomic changes in animals and biochemical changes in the central nervous system. They believe that these changes correlate with the improvement in seizures, paresis (impaired movement), and paralysis treated with acupuncture. Vagus nerve stimulation (VNS) and neurotransmitter changes explain the effects of acupuncture on the brain on epilepsy. This is also the biochemical mechanism of VNS. Acupuncture points on the body, face, ear, scalp, and lower extremities activate the vagus nerve through reflex actions taking place in centers that receive several converging inputs within the brain stem. These points appear frequently in treating epilepsy.

Bob Flaws, an internationally acclaimed practitioner, author, and teacher of Chinese medicine, has written an important book on treating brain illness with acupuncture. Herbal formulas to treat epilepsy can be found in another book by noted teacher, herbalist, and author Dr. Honora Wolfe of Boulder, Colorado. Her Blue Poppy Herb website offers their Chinese medicine and herbal books. Blue Poppy Herb's laboratory tested herbal formulas can be purchased solely by an acupuncturist or medical doctor. Dr. John and Tina Chen, LAc of California have also written a comprehensive herbal book for Chinese medicine single herbs.

Acupuncture is a wonderful tool for treating seizure disorders and epilepsy. The brain's excess electrical activity often has an imbalance of hormones or neurotransmitters. Herbs and acupuncture can reduce these imbalances. Three types of acupuncture can treat seizures: scalp, auricular, and body acupuncture. It would be wise to initially avoid electro-stim with the acupuncture. Acupuncture will not cure epilepsy in a single session. Retention needles - small needles that can be left in place after the session - may be useful in many cases. A special French technique is able to reduce excess electrical activity more quickly, but it is not widely available and is more expensive.

Auricular acupuncture points that have improved seizures or epilepsy include the epilepsy point, brain stem, shen men, brain, heart, occiput, liver, endocrine, cortex, subcortex, and large intestine.

Shen men is an acupuncture point on the ear that has received extensive examination. Its location on the ear lies within the zone of the concave surface of the pinna, supplied by the auricular branch of the vagus nerve. Electro-acupuncture is electrical stimulation applied to an acupuncture needle. Auricular electro-acupuncture stimulation decreases epileptic activity in the cortex of the brain. Electro-acupuncture decreases levels of excitatory neurotransmitters in the hippocampus and increases the inhibitory neurotransmitter levels of glycine, taurine, and GABA. Quantum Brain Healing has found herbal formulas and acupuncture to successfully reduce and stop seizures. Always discuss with your practitioner any new medications or recreational drugs that are being used, as these may trigger seizures in some people. You *must* examine medication use when seizures commence.

Stimulation of acupuncture points on the extremities results in stimulation of the vagus nerve. The anti-epileptic effects of VNS and electro-acupuncture target the same part of the brain. Taurine supplementation increases the effectiveness of electro-acupuncture to protect against induced seizures. Some Chinese herbs used to treat epilepsy have relatively high amounts of taurine.

Electro-acupuncture applied to body points in rats with pilocarpine-induced epilepsy levels found that electro-acupuncture reduced epileptiform discharges in the improved cognitive deficits and prevented shrinkage of areas within the limbic system of the brain. Electro-acupuncture functions as a neuroprotectant. It is likely that acupuncture and electro-acupuncture reverse signs of brain aging and mental decline. The brain can make new neural networks, and nutritional support and acupuncture are key to this process. The addition of alpha lipoic acid, omega-3 essential acids, and choline may speed the establishment of new neural network interconnections and can be taken one hour prior to the treatment.

The use of organic products and organic food is very important, as is minimizing toxic household cleaning items and improving air quality with an ionizing household air filter. Focus on avoiding commonly encountered pesticides, such as dieldrin, lindane and the pyrethroids, which interfere with the brain's electrical activity of the brain. Pesticides and other toxins can bind with benzodiazepine receptors and cause seizures or convulsions in some people. Energy disruption through exposure to excess electromagnetic fields can cause seizures in susceptible people. Try to avoid areas where there are too many cell phone towers and wireless systems in one place.

Heavy metal toxins such as lead, mercury, cadmium, titanium, and aluminum interfere with proper nerve function and can cause seizures or convulsions. Dental amalgam contains mercury which crosses the blood brain barrier. This alters brain activity and neurotransmitters levels. Research studies show that epilepsy can improve after removal of dental amalgam.

Herbs

Quantum Brain Healing uses several Chinese patent formulas to treat or heal seizures and epilepsy. These formulas include:

> **Tian Ma Gou Teng Yin,** or Gastrodia and Unicaria Formula

> **Ding Xian Wan**, or Stopping Epilepsy Pill; Arrest Seizures Pill; Gastrodia and

Succinum Pill

> **Wu Sheng Jia Er Chen Tang,** or Five-Fresh and Two-Cured Decoction

> **Er Zhi Xian Fang,** or Ultimate Immortals

There are many great single herbs that are affordable and easily found in most vitamin stores. They may be tried one at a time to determine which one has the most impact on your seizure disorder. For example, gastrodia is frequently tried for healing the brain, along with other nutritional support. This herb is also referred to as Tian Ma in Traditional Chinese Medicine. It is safe enough to be used on young children and infants. It can be safely used with many other herbs. It is used in Orthomolecular Medicine with high doses of vitamins, minerals, and nutritional supplements to treat very complex diseases.

This herb is used to protect the brain and keep brain cells from dying. It enhances the mitochondria's ability to produce energy. This herb has a sedative effect. Gastrodia lowers blood pressure and can be used to treat hypertensive headaches and migraine headaches. It would be safe to try on a preventive basis during periods where there are several migraine headaches during a week.

Gastrodia protects the brain from seizures and convulsions. This herb can be taken by those suffering from non-defined seizures and some types of epilepsy. Gastrodia can be used for acute or chronic infantile convulsions and seizures, but this must be done under the care of a health care professional and very closely followed for changes in sleep patterns, seizure behavior patterns, the frequency of seizures or convulsions, how long the seizures last, and eating patterns of the child. If the seizures occur less frequently and last for a longer time period after starting on gastrodia, this herb should be discontinued immediately. If the seizures drastically shorten in time and occur slightly more often, the dosage of the herb may need to be adjusted. For extremely difficult diseases, the exact dosage of the herb may be difficult to find.

This herb has an anti-inflammatory effect, and this may be part of the action in preventing seizures. Gastrodia can be used for treating Huntington's disease. Allow one to four weeks before adjusting the dosage of this herb for Huntington's. Huntington's disease requires very high levels of vitamins and branched amino acids to support the overall health. An organic diet without refined foods is best for someone with Huntington's. Make sure that there are adequate levels of unsaturated fatty acids to facilitate recovery and treatment of any brain disease.

Quantum Brain Healing also utilizes the skullcap herb for many brain diseases that require calming or sedating a part of the brain. Skullcap and Orthomolecular Medicine may be useful in speeding the balancing of neurotransmitter levels. Most brain diseases are rooted in the basis of unbalanced neurotransmitters. Amino acids can quickly rebalance the neurotransmitter levels when the correct ones are chosen and the correct ratio of amino acids is used. This is difficult to achieve for those medical professionals without experience in Orthomolecular Medicine. Scutellaria lateriflora, or the skullcap leaf, has sedative, anticonvulsive and anti-inflammatory effects on the brain. This herb has been used in America for hundreds of years; this is not a Chinese herb.

Skullcap may be used to treat brain disease including epilepsy, ADD, headaches, neuralgia, insomnia, hysteria, anxiety, delirium, and convulsions. Skullcap can be used in addiction disorders for symptoms like withdrawal from barbiturates, alcohol, and tranquilizers.

Quantum Brain Healing combines therapeutic doses of amino acids, vitamins, minerals, nutritional supplements, and herbs to treat or heal many brain diseases. This may heal the disease, treat the disease, or reduce the amount of a drug. Vinpocetine is an herbal extract that is derived from the periwinkle plant. This herbal extract has many properties that make it important in healing the brain. This extract crosses blood-brain barrier and acts as a neuroprotectant to protect the brain cells and keep them alive longer.

Vinpocetine is an antioxidant that improves brain circulation and metabolism. It can be used to protect the brain for patients who are subject to strokes and ischemia. After a patient has a stroke, this extract can be useful in protecting brain cells in the event of a future attack. The extract acts as an anticonvulsant and antismolytic. The anticonvulsant action allows it to reduce seizures in some and prevent seizures in others. This also delays the decline for many Alzheimer's patients. It can prevent atherosclerosis when taken on a long-term basis. It slows or prevents abnormal platelet clumping. This is considered an anti-aging brain supplement. It should not be used by those taking blood thinners, nor should it be taken with large quantities of green tea, as vinpocetine has blood-thinning properties.

Vinpocetine can be useful for many people in treating seizures, as well as ischemia, dementia, Alzheimer's disease, Parkinson's disease, and memory loss. Vinpocetine may be useful in treating epilepsy caused by traumatic injury. This treatment would be best when tried within one to six months after the injury and would need to be combined with other Quantum Brain Healing therapy.

Quantum Brain Healing uses many amino acids, vitamins, minerals, nutritional supplements, and herbs to treat and help improve brain diseases. Jack-in-the-pulpit is one of the least used and most complicated herbs- it is seldom prescribed due to its strong medical properties—but this herb can *only be used under the care of a health care professional.* Do not ever use this herb by yourself; it cannot ever be viewed as an herb to purchase online or in an herb shop.

Jack-in-the-pulpit is also referred to as Tian Nan Xing in Traditional Chinese Medicine. It has analgesic and sedative medical properties. It acts as an anti-inflammatory agent in the brain. It can be used to treat seizures and convulsions. Never use this type of herb on a patient who is unable to communicate with the family or doctors. It would be very easy to overdose this type of patient. Do not use this herb on a young child or combine this herb with other herbs during its initial trial use.

Quantum Brain Healing uses Jack-in-the-pulpit to treat convulsions, seizures, paralysis, spasms, stroke, dizziness, ischemia, epilepsy, and peripheral neuralgia. This herb may have a negative impact on the heart and kidneys of extremely weak and older patients. In cases of paralysis and epilepsy, however, it may be advisable for some people to have this herbal option. The patient must not drink alcohol or use recreational drugs when taking this herb. A good balanced diet is also needed.

If I were a person recently paralyzed, I would want a doctor to try this on me before I gave up. Good health before any of these illnesses strike is a prerequisite for trying Jack-in-the-pulpit, but to use it, the patient needs to locate an Orthomolecular Medicine doctor or acupuncturist who specializes in herbal medicine.

Vitamins

Quantum Brain Healing treats epilepsy by analyzing the root of the disease. Triggers of epilepsy include vitamin and mineral deficiencies, food allergies, stress, environmental toxins and allergens, physical or emotional trauma, neurotoxins like aspartame, allergic reactions to pharmaceutical drugs, recreational drug abuse, stimulants, sleep deprivation, strobe light exposure, low blood sugar, extreme temperature exposure (either hot or cold), trauma, and dehydration.

Many types of illness can produce seizures in a crisis stage. Although uncommon, a diabetic patient whose glucose levels are extremely low or high may experience a seizure. Diabetic patients must have their glucose levels stabilized to avoid seizures. (This event would be a seizure disorder rather than epilepsy.) Detoxification will benefit many patients react to toxins and allergens. Detox can shorten or eliminate some seizures.

One-half of epileptic patients have abnormal carbohydrate metabolism, resulting in hypoglycemia. Low blood sugar can trigger a seizure or cause the person to faint. Eating can stave off a seizure if the epileptic person closely monitors symptoms of hypoglycemia. The epileptic patient often has low levels of vitamin B1, vitamin B6, calcium, manganese, zinc, and magnesium, and they are often deficient in L-cysteine. Quantum Brain Healing will replace the missing nutrients in therapeutic doses.

Electrical activity of the brain is affected by the excess or deficiency of nutritional factors including vitamins, minerals, and phytonutrients. Seizures can be caused by deficiencies of vitamin B-3 or vitamin B-6. Extremely excessive levels of vitamin A also can result in seizures. Quantum Brain Healing uses amino acid therapy along with nutritional supplements to restore the brain to its non-seizure state. Acupuncture can be used to rewire the brain. When the correct supplements are used with acupuncture, new brain cells can grow, and the brain can slowly be rewired for some people. Children who are born with epilepsy are more difficult to treat. It is difficult to treat patients who are unable to communicate.

Nutritional Supplements

Nutritional supplements that treat or improve epilepsy or seizures include PS (phosphatidylserine), omega-3 fatty acids (fish oil), lithium orotate, vitamin B-6, folate, niacin, SOD (superoxide dismutase), NAC (N-acetylcysteine), melatonin, and vinpocetine.

Orthomolecular Medicine

Quantum Brain Healing uses several amino acids in treating seizures and epilepsy. These include taurine, DMG, GABA, and DMG. It may require more than one amino acid to treat the disease, and therapeutic doses are administered. These sizable doses of amino acids will need to be taken for three years. This is affected by whether the herbal formulas are being taken simultaneously. GABA is an amino acid and a neurotransmitter that can be effective in treating epilepsy, schizophrenia, and other brain disorders.

Taurine is a neurotransmitter and a modulator of neurotransmission. It impacts neural pathway function and has a role in epilepsy. Research demonstrates that taurine reduces seizures in some patients. In one small study, nine patients were treated with taurine (100 mg/kgm/day) or a placebo for two months. Using taurine supplementation, one patient had nearly complete cessation of seizures, and two patients decreased seizure activity by about half. Liquid taurine supplementation will produce better results for most people.

It is possible that the use of dietary enzymes would have increased the success of this clinical trial. Impaired digestive tracts have a large impact on the absorption level of any substance. Taurine does not easily cross the blood-brain barrier, but I believe in the future it will be utilized as a mainline treatment for epilepsy by combining it with a nontoxic carrier that enables safe passage into the brain in an IV form. Many herbs can be safely used for this purpose. I would alter the choice of the carrier herb, depending upon the other symptoms of the patient.

DMG, or dimethylglycine, is a derivative of the amino acid glycine. It is also known as vitamin B-15 in Russia. Russia uses this to treat drug addiction, alcoholism, autism, schizophrenia, children with minimal brain damage, senile dementia, and cognitive impairment.

Beans, cereal grains, and liver contain significant amounts of DMG. DMG is an antioxidant and immune enhancer, and it increases brain oxygen levels. It is produced in cells during the metabolism of choline. DMG has been used to treat epilepsy, seizures, and autism. It will not cure the disease but may reduce the frequency of the seizures.

Diet

Quantum Brain Healing may try several different types of diets to stop or diminish the severity of seizures. The diet may take five weeks to show progress. Other diets available include the rotation diet, the elimination diet, and the ketogenic diet, which can resolve or diminish seizures. Many seizures can be triggered by food allergies or environmental toxins.

The glutamate-aspartate restricted diet (GARD) is a type of elimination diet developed to treat epilepsy in animals. It identifies foods and ingredients that should be avoided, including the following:

- gluten found in wheat and grains
- casein in protein found in cow's milk and dairy products
- soy
- corn, including corn syrup and corn derivative products
- MSG (monosodium glutamate)
- aspartame (Nutra Sweet) used as a sugar substitute
- glutamate found in high concentrations in most beans/legumes
- hydrogenated oils

The GARD is a glutamate-aspartate restricted diet due to the limitation of these two nonessential, neurostimulating amino acids that are also the parent compounds of MSG and aspartame (NutraSweet). Aspartame is a neurotoxin that has been connected with brain cancer in Italy. Glutamate and aspartate are excitotoxins. They are able to trigger seizures

134

and cause neurodegenerative diseases in some patients. The GARD is also referred to as the "gut absorption recovery diet," due to its removal of gluten, dairy, soy, and corn. These foods may induce damage to the intestinal villi, resulting in celiac disease and food intolerance.

There is anecdotal evidence that this diet works to eliminate or reduce seizures for people diagnosed with mesial temporal lobe epilepsy (MTLE) and atrophy of the hippocampus. There is little or no published clinical research for GARD. If effective, this diet needs to be adopted as a permanent lifestyle change. It requires continuous active participation to maintain seizure control. Seizure control can occur very quickly, within several weeks, with this diet. GARD is the only "seizure control" diet that does not restrict carbohydrate consumption. It allows high-glycemic and high-carbohydrates foods. Diabetics, hypoglycemics or anyone who has sensitivity to dietary sugars should try GARD only under the strict supervision of their doctor. Patients with diseases that result in or cause atrophy of the hippocampus should try this diet or another diet that eliminates dietary glutamate. GARD might be good for a Parkinson's patient.

Quantum Brain Healing usually requires nutritional changes to manage epilepsy and seizure disorder. The diet always impacts the course of any disease. Seizures triggered by food allergies will diminish after the food trigger is identified. The ketogenic diet is a good diet to try if other therapies are unable to improve the disease.

The ketogenic diet is a high-fat, low-carbohydrate diet, with a moderate to high amount of protein. It can be used to treat epilepsy, but it is not an overnight fix. It can moderate electrical activity in the brain if used more than two years. This is a difficult diet, as it produces an effect similar to starvation and forces the body to burn fat instead of carbohydrates. Calories are strictly controlled so that weight is not lost or gained during the diet. Regular growth and repair of the body continues. The ketogenic diet is heavily supplemented with vitamins and minerals. It should be done under the care of a registered dietician or physician. Fluids are restricted so that electrolytes do not get out of balance.

The ketogenic diet seems to alter the seizure threshold with the elevation of ketone levels. When glucose is insufficient, the body burns fat. The fat is not completely burned, however, and ketones are formed. The high level of ketones formed seems to reduce or eliminate seizures in many people. People who are unable to control seizure activity by other means can use this diet. They should discontinue this diet after they have been seizure-free for a period of approximately two years. In 1998, Johns Hopkins Medical School released a study on the ketogenic diet, which showed the diet significantly helped eliminate the seizure activity in approximately one-third of the patients studied. Other patients showed reduced seizure activity.

In 2005, Emory University School of Medicine showed that this diet alters the genes involved in energy metabolism of the brain. This action helps to stabilize neurons when seizure activity occurs. The ketogenic diet increased the energy production in the hippocampus, helped the brain to become more resistant to reduced glucose levels, and increased the brain's ability to handle metabolism changes.

Side effects of the ketogenic diet include dehydration, kidney stones, constipation, vomiting, increased cholesterol, lower growth rate, behavior changes, and mood changes. There are other diets to try if this diet is unsuccessful.

Nutrition

The zinc and copper ratio is often out of balance for many people with epilepsy - the zinc level is low and copper level is high. This ratio needs to be addressed with close monitoring. Dietary changes focusing on eating more foods high in zinc or taking zinc supplementation may be necessary.

The following foods are believed by some to have value in reducing the frequency seizures: asparagus, beans, liver, carob, wheat, white lupine, Chinese cabbage, soybean, chives, buffalo gourd, groundnut, grains, butternut, almond, opium poppy, tomato, Italian stone pine, chaya, cowpea, black beans, pignut hickory, and white mustard. Their ability to have this biochemical action likely is in their chemical and nutritional structure.

Hyperbaric Oxygen Therapy

This is a type of oxygen therapy where patients breathe pure oxygen in a chamber with a higher-than-normal atmospheric pressure. This is reported to have successful results in treating some cases of epilepsy. This has been also used to treat carbon monoxide poisoning, viral-based pulmonary diseases, multiple sclerosis, dementia, cognitive impairment, stroke rehabilitation, and traumatic brain injury.

Aromatherapy

Dr. Tim Betts at Queen Elizabeth Hospital in Birmingham, England, researched aromatherapy as a means to help to control epilepsy. Some people with seizures get a warning that includes seeing an aura prior to its onset and may be able to breathe in the scent of aromatic oils at the start of the warning to reduce the severity or occurrence of the epileptic seizure. This should be carefully done under the guidance of a professional due to the fact that some essential oils - such as wormwood, sage, rosemary, hyssop, and fennel actually can trigger seizures in epileptics and should be avoided.

Homeopathy

There is little published clinical research outside the Europe that examines the effectiveness of specific homeopathic remedies. Professional homeopaths recommend one or more treatments for seizure disorders, based on their knowledge and clinical experience. Homeopaths take into account a person's constitutional type when deciding a treatment plan. In homeopathic terms, a person's constitution is his or her physical, emotional, and intellectual makeup. An experienced homeopath assesses all of these factors when determining the most appropriate remedy for a particular individual.

At least four homeopathic remedies are able to help some types of epilepsy. Belladonna treats seizures that occur in individuals with a high fever. Causticum treats individuals whose seizures may be triggered by receiving bad news or by feelings of sadness, such as from grief - this remedy is most appropriate for individuals who tend to feel hopeless and fearful. Cicuta treats individuals who develop seizures after a head injury. Cuprum metallicum treats individuals whose seizures are accompanied by mental dullness and which may be triggered by menstruation or vomiting.

Reflexology

Quantum Brain Healing uses many vitamins, minerals, amino acids, and herbs to treat epilepsy, but many additional alternative therapies in Quantum Brain Healing are used to treat epilepsy, including reflexology.

Reflexology is based on the principle that the anatomy of the body is reflected in miniature reflex zones on the head, ears, hands and feet. The foot is the most common type of reflexology treatment, where pressure is applied on the foot to heal the body. Reflexology promotes relaxation and reduces stress. Both feet are worked on during the course of a full session.

The reflexologist will gently massage your feet and apply pressure to the reflex points that correlate to your health problems. With epilepsy, there would be pressure applied to the head, brain, brain stem, pituitary, pineal/hypothalamus, thyroid, parathyroid, and adrenal glands areas. This concept is similar to the concept of acupressure. Some reflexologists apply pressure with their fingers, while others use small instruments.

People with foot problems, such as severe calluses or corns, should visit a podiatrist for treatment prior to a reflexology treatment. Sessions typically last sixty minutes. Epilepsy is usually a chronic disease and would require many treatments. Many reflexologists believe that manipulation of the feet reduces the lactic acid accumulation in the tissues and releases tiny calcium crystals that accumulate in the nerve endings of the feet. Another way to reinforce this action on the feet is to purchase an infrared foot massager. Foot ionizing detoxification may also help remove calcium and lactic acid build up from your feet.

Reflexology restores the qi, or free flow of energy, from the feet to the corresponding organs. Some reflexologists believe that pressure on the reflex points may trigger the release of hormones, including endorphins, chemicals in the brain that naturally block pain. Reflexology creates relaxation, improves circulation, and increases the rate at which detoxification occurs. Reflexology can help control seizures for some patients, but there are no major clinical research trials to verify the effectiveness of reflexology with epilepsy patients. Reflexology should be used in addition to other therapies.

Emotional Freedom Technique (EFT)

Emotional Freedom Technique, or EFT, is a therapy which excels at treating symptoms related to emotions. Seizures may be reduced with EFT. This therapy benefits people with disease and emotional trauma. It could alter the electro-magnetic field of the patient.

EFT uses fingers to perform a tapping motion on acupuncture points along energy meridians established in Traditional Chinese Medicine. This is known as EFT tapping. The points that are tapped must be exactly correct in location. There may be additional points added to your treatment, depending upon your specific injury, disease, or level of emotional distress. This technique must usually be done more than once in order for it to succeed. Positive and negative affirmations are stated out loud while the tapping is done.

This therapy can alter your thought and feelings. Many diseases can improve and heal when the person changes his beliefs about getting well. EFT tapping may be able to move the blocked energy along Chinese energy meridians and alter feelings. There are several energy meridians in the body, and they correspond to specific organs.

When the body's energy gets blocked or stuck in a specific organ, like the heart or small intestine, it may impact several organs and energy throughout the entire body. Chinese medicine believes that each energy meridian and organ is connected to emotions, directly or indirectly. As energetic blockages are removed and the energy flows freely, the person will improve the symptom and any emotionally caused problems can heal. It is possible for a person to get well in a single treatment. Many people will require several sessions.

EFT can be used for healing seizures and tics. It is not a cure for epilepsy; rather, it can improve the seizures associated with stress, anxiety, or depression. It can reduce the

138

emotional component of epilepsy or seizure disorders. It is important to differentiate between seizures and epilepsy.

Music Therapy

Quantum Brain Healing relies on adjunct therapies will be used for very hard cases. Metatones is auditory vibrational energy therapy to address problems for epilepsy, learning disabilities, dyslexia, and insomnia. Auditory therapy can indirectly affect neurotransmitter levels. Hormones are one factor that can impact the severity in seizures. Hormone therapy may be a great idea to combine with music therapy for older patients if their hormones are low. This therapy is effective for those with seizures of an unknown origin. This therapy is always better from a trained music therapist.

Music therapy, Acutonics (sound healing education), singing, and Tibetan singing bowls are simpler versions of the concept of using music or sound vibrations to heal. The Hemi-Sync method is a more sophisticated version of vibrational sound therapy developed by Dr. Robert Monroe. The brain can be balanced by auditory therapy. The sounds are played on a CD and listened to with headphones. The brain-wave activity is altered by the sound vibration as it is heard. There are several types of brain waves, and your brain may not experience proper brain-wave activity. The Hemi-Sync method adjusts the brain-wave activity.

Research shows that brains of Parkinson's and Alzheimer's patients have decidedly different brain waves than the normal brain. Hemi-Sync works to entrain the brain into the proper brain-wave activity for health. Vibrational energy healing is based on the tenet that disease stems from a lack of proper resonance. Music therapy and sound therapy have many successful results. Most forms of medicine believe that disease is rooted by a lack of balance. Hemi-Sync can be used for many years to help balance your brain.

Health will return when cells are put into vibrational balance. Music therapy may be one more way to influence and change neurotransmitter levels. Classical music and baroque music are the best music for balancing the brain. Music therapy with a harp has been used to treat MS. Learning to play the piano or guitar can help balance the brain of a child with ADD or ADHD. Singing upbeat songs is a great way for a child to improve their depression. Stroke patients that are unable to speak may be able to hum along with music.

Vagus Nerve Stimulation (VNS)

Medicine understands that there is no single answer to good health. It is key to remain open to technology when other options have not met our goals. One option that can be considered after trying nutritional therapy is vagus nerve stimulation (VNS), an option that must be sought through a surgeon—this is a medical device (a flat, round battery, similar to a pacemaker and about the size of a silver dollar) that is surgically implanted. Most insurers cover the cost of the device and the surgery for implantation. Any major medical center in the United States and Europe can implant this device for a patient who qualifies.

The vagus nerve is part of the autonomic nervous system and controls involuntary body functions. Vagus nerve stimulation (VNS) involves sending a message to the brain using periodic, mild electrical stimulation from the vagus nerve in the neck. There is no brain surgery involved. VNS may control epilepsy in cases where anti-epileptic drugs are ineffective or have intolerable side effects or when neurosurgery is not appropriate. VNS is effective in stopping seizures in some patients. Contact Dr. Heidi Seifert of the Seifert Pain Clinic in Houston for more information on this procedure and whether it is an option for you. Dr. Heidi Seifert is a splendid pain doctor. You can also contact Dr. Chuck Brunacardi with Baylor in the Texas Medical Center. Mayo Clinic is another healthcare provider for this surgery with locations in Minnesota, Arizona, and Florida.

The doctor determines the strength and timing of the pulses administered by the device, according to each patient's individual needs. The level of electrical stimulation can be changed without additional surgery with a programming wand connected to a laptop computer.

The side effects of VNS during treatment may include hoarseness, coughing, throat pain, shortness of breath, a short and slight sensation of choking, altered voice sound, ear pain, tooth pain, and a tingling sensation in the neck. Skin irritation or infection could occur at the implantation site. VNS does not negatively impact the brain. This is major surgery and should not be considered lightly. Consider all options before giving up on controlling seizure. For those with uncontrollable epileptic seizures, it may be a last option. VNS is safer than neurosurgery.

Those with epilepsy should strongly consider the following:

- Avoid recreational drugs
- Be very careful around gasoline fumes at filling stations
- Go indoors to avoid any type of explosion where a gas is released
- Use caution when taking over-the counter medicines
- Inform your doctor of all medications that you are taking
- Avoid mold and mildew
- Use extra caution with cleaning products that have fumes like Clorox, oven

cleaners, dry cleaning products, and ammonia

People with epilepsy also should avoid brain-stimulating substances of all types, including the following:

- ➤ Alcohol
- ➤ Cocaine
- ➤ Amphetamines
- ➤ Evening primrose oil
- ➤ Tyrosine
- ➤ Ephedra
- ➤ Caffeine (coffee or tea)
- ➤ Guarana
- ➤ Citrus aurantium
- ➤ Ginkgo
- ➤ Horny goat weed
- ➤ DMAE
- ➤ 5-HTP

INSOMNIA

Quantum Brain Healing uses many therapies to heal insomnia. People taking medicine for other health problems make want to start with the yoga and qi gong. Medical devices such as biofeedback, acupuncture, and the Bio-Mat are also great for people taking medicine. There is no chemical interaction with your medicine when using this approach. Vitamins and minerals are the next addition in your protocol to solve insomnia. Chinese herbal medicines and botanical extracts are wonderful and can be implemented for further solutions.

Insomnia should be analyzed to determine its organic causes. Hormone imbalance, marital stress, job uncertainty, high workload, and viral or bacterial infections all could cause insomnia. It is often a side effect of many types of drug and alcohol addiction. The person with insomnia should be tested and blood work should be evaluated for bacterial or viral infections.

Insomnia causes stress to become worse. Diabetes may get worse, and you may have higher glucose levels. Any bacterial infection gets worse when you are exhausted due to lack of sleep. Car-accident rates rise during times of insomnia. You are less likely to take good care of yourself. You may consume a poor diet and overeat. Your sex life might suffer. Drug use increases during insomnia and high-stress periods. Viral infections may increase drastically. You may be too tired to exercise. You may forget to take vitamins. You might drink too much caffeine. You might push yourself very hard and compensate with stimulants, like coffee.

Severe sleep deprivation caused by hormone deficiencies may cause depression. The hormone imbalances can be corrected with bio-identical hormones or Chinese herbal patent formulas. Chinese patent formulas will take approximately two to five weeks for the full extent of their benefits to be viewed, relative to hormone changes. Depression can lift of its own accord when these issues are managed. Another causative factor for insomnia may be anxiety, bipolar disorder, or mania diseases.

Try to develop a safe haven to sleep, where no TV or other activities are allowed. Do not work or eat in your bedroom. Your sleep environment should include cotton, silk, or wool products on the bed. The Sharper Image's air ionizing machine can improve air-quality issues. An ionizing filtration system for the air conditioning and heating unit for the entire household may be beneficial. Sleep might be interrupted due to heat or cold. Install a ceiling fan, and make sure there are adequate blankets on the bed. The successful management of insomnia can go a very long way toward improving your energy levels.

Amino Acid Therapy

Orthomolecular Medicine can be used to treat insomnia. The amino acids used can include 5-HTP, theanine, GABA, and orthinine.

GABA is an amino acid used in the field of holistic healing to treat insomnia, depression, and anxiety. It may be very effective for those people who cannot use antidepressants due to side effects. GABA is an amino acid that is a calming neurotransmitter. A shortage of GABA can prevent you from falling asleep or cause you to wake-up in the middle of the night. It can also cause you to sleep lightly and wake up more easily. It is usually deficient in those with depression and anxiety. There are frequently several neurotransmitters imbalances in most brain diseases.

Another amino acid that is used in Orthomolecular Medicine is 5-HTP. This supplement can be used to calm overstimulated or overexcited nerves. This amino acid can also replace tricyclic antidepressants used in the treatment of neuropathy in some cases. 5-HTP may be used at higher doses to treat overeating related to mood disorders and depression—this would be for a mild to moderate case. Extremely severe cases may not be able to use this treatment protocol to replace drug therapy. It may be useful in serious cases to lower the amount of the drug required by the patient.

Quantum Brain Healing uses melatonin to help treat depression along with amino acids, vitamins, minerals, and herbs. Melatonin is a hormone produced in the brain by the pineal gland from the amino acid tryptophan. It is available as a nutritional supplement. You can also increase melatonin levels by supplementing the amino acid tryptophan. Melatonin is stimulated by darkness and suppressed by light and is affected by the circadian rhythm. It regulates diverse body functions. Levels of melatonin in the blood are highest prior to bedtime. Low levels of melatonin are associated with some types of cancer.

Melatonin may help treat depression that stems from inadequate sleep. When the sleep cycle is improved, this type of depression patient will often recover quickly. Melatonin is a good supplement to take at night thirty minutes before bedtime to help you fall asleep. It can improve the quality of your sleep. It is important to refrain from high doses of this supplement and use a supplement from 1 to 4 mg/ day. Anxiety is also a problem when there is sleep deprivation. Almost every type of brain condition gets worse when there is insufficient sleep. It is important to ask your doctor about this problem. Hormone imbalances often cause many brain conditions during menopause or andropause.

Melatonin will cross the blood-brain barrier and increase brain circulation. It increases the production of neurotransmitters and balances the brain. It strengthens the immune system.

The enhanced immune system is due to the improvement in hormone and neurotransmitter regulation.

Quantum Brain Healing uses melatonin to treat insomnia, jet lag, ischemia, smoking cessation, sleep disturbances related to depression, depression caused by sleep deprivation, seasonal affective disorder (SAD), and anxiety. This hormone may be combined with amino acids to increase its effectiveness. Nutritional support can include food based multivitamins, vitamin E, vitamin D, CoQ10, and alpha lipoic acid. Try adding yoga or mild exercise for producing maximum results from melatonin.

If there is a melatonin deficiency, the body's circadian rhythm is imbalanced, and the body will wake up at irregular times due to brain-wave irregularities and hormone imbalances. Melatonin supplements of 1.5 to 3 mg per day, taken for about four weeks, may help this deficiency. A combination capsule containing vitamin D, magnesium, and calcium is another aid for sleep. St. John's wort, hops, valerian, passionflower, chamomile, and lemon balm are herbs that may induce sleep. Bach Flower Remedies are a wonderful, mild tool for helping people relax and can treat insomnia. Aromatic essential oils are also a great tool - small pillows filled with lavender can be warmed in the microwave to release the aroma.

Bio-Identical Hormones

Bio-identical hormones may help treat insomnia caused by hormone imbalances due to menopause and andropause for people aged forty to seventy. Insomnia is a huge problem for many menopausal women. Hot flashes may wake the woman, but neurotransmitter and glucose swings also cause insomnia. Bio-identical progesterone may help balance the hormones for women during or nearing menopause. Men can also use androgen and testosterone bio-identical hormones to help them prevent memory loss and concentration issues. Amino acids, vitamins, food, single herbs like horny goat weed and vitex, and patent herbal formulas are able to increase hormone and neurotransmitters levels.

DHEA

DHEA is a natural hormone precursor to estrogen and androgen produced from cholesterol. Your body's own DHEA levels may be reduced by taking insulin, corticosteroids, opiates, or danazol. Twenty percent of Americans have a DHEA deficiency.

DHEA improves mood and acts as an anti-inflammatory and immunity booster. This can be taken with a probiotic capsule for increased absorption rates in some people.

It is anti-aging antioxidant that can decrease evening cortisol levels. Its ability to reduce cortisol levels is how it can help with insomnia. It can also benefit those with anxiety, depression, memory loss, and dementia. It may be used in treating Alzheimer's and ischemia.

Vitamins

Vitamin B12 can help balance neurotransmitters and treat insomnia. Vitamin B12 is involved in DNA synthesis and fatty acid synthesis, and it helps break down carbohydrates and convert them into energy. It is used by the body to help make several amino acids, including SAM-e. These amino acids are found to change brain chemistry and neurotransmitter levels. The neurotransmitters affected by vitamin B12 directly are involved in learning skills and memory. A sub-lingual form of B12 is far more absorbable form. A multivitamin product should also be taken with this supplement so that the other B vitamins do not become deficient.

Symptoms of vitamin B12 deficiency include fatigue, brain fog, delusion, poor memory, neurological problems, poor concentration, depression, psychosis, irritability, mania, forgetfulness, and increased sleep requirements. These symptoms also could be indicative of other vitamin or mineral deficiencies. Any of the above conditions may be treated with vitamin B12 if a deficiency exists. When there are multiple vitamin deficiencies, all must be treated for the patient to heal.

Quantum Orthomolecular Medicine uses higher amounts of vitamin B12 than would be found in a multivitamin product or normal diet. Many brain diseases may require these higher levels of vitamin B12 in order for healing to occur. Diseases improved by taking vitamin B12 include Alzheimer's disease, dementia, depression, long-term memory loss, and impaired ability to convert short-term memory into long-term memory. The brain fog symptom associated with chronic fatigue syndrome can be improved with increased doses of this supplement. It is always worth noting that digestive problems may be the root of vitamin deficiencies. A digestive enzyme might allow you to better absorb most of your vitamins. Vitamin B12 is found in beef, caviar, chicken, cheese, eggs, fish, lamb, liver, milk, octopus, and shellfish.

Choline is brain food. CDP-choline is a form of choline and cytidine. Choline is a precursor to phosphatidylcholine (PS). It is used in the structure and function of cells. It is a precursor to acetylcholine. CDP-choline can affect many neurological functions. Its actions include crossing blood-brain barrier, acting as an antioxidant, and acting as an cognitive enhancer. It is an immune enhancer, neuroprotectant, and cyto-protectant. It improves neurological function in an overstressed person. It helps balance the brain, and this action improves insomnia.

Herbs

Quantum Brain Healing uses kava kava to sedate the overactive brain. Kava acts on the limbic system, and it affects several neurotransmitters, including GABA and noradrenalin. The limbic area of the brain is key to your emotions of sadness, fear, and anger.

Kava has anticonvulsant effects. It is an anti-inflammatory and can be considered a secondary level anti-aging herb. It can act as a muscle relaxant on the skeletal muscles and central nervous system. Kava is an anxiolytic and may be used to treat anxiety. Kava can enhance cognitive thinking skills and improve reaction time. It is important not to overuse this herb.

It may be an adaptogen due to its slight ability to elevate mood and sedate. Frequently, herbs that can produce two opposing actions, depending upon what is needed by the body, are considered adaptogens. Taking kava is associated with lower levels of leukemia and ovarian cancer, according to a study at the University of Aberdeen in Scotland. It is important to note that there are reports by a few of severe liver toxicity from this herb. This may be due to problems with how it is made or other substances that the patients are consuming while on kava.

Kava can be used to treat anxiety, nervousness, stress, and insomnia. These conditions are related for many people, and the slight sedating effect that kava has may resolve anxiety and stress. This may be the mechanism of how the insomnia is resolved. Kava also treats agoraphobia; this may be tied to its ability to affect the limbic area of the brain.

Kava must be supported with vitamins, minerals, and high levels of antioxidants. A break should be taken from this herb after you have taken it to seven weeks on a regular basis. The break should last for at least ten to twelve days. Eat a wide variety of organic vegetables and fruits, and avoid alcohol, cigarettes, nicotine, and recreational drugs when taking kava. Do not overload the liver with toxins from eating a diet high in refined foods, alcohol, recreational drugs, or over the counter drugs. A regular liver detoxification is a good idea for anyone taking this herb.

Kava is not recommended for those with Parkinson's, liver disease, lung disease, depression, or bipolar disorder. Kava has negative interactions with acetazolamide, amiloride, furosemide, or with angiotensin-converting enzyme (ACE) inhibitors such as benazepril, captopril, lisinopril, quinapril, ramipril, levodopa-based medication, alcohol, Xanax, barbiturates, or other mood-altering drugs.

Skullcap may be used to treat brain disease, including insomnia, epilepsy, ADD, headaches, neuralgia, hysteria, anxiety, delirium, and convulsions. Skullcap can be used in addiction disorders for withdrawal from barbiturates, alcohol, and tranquilizers. Preventing brain disease and protecting the brain is an important step in your anti-aging program. Adequate sleep can help control weight, stabilize moods, and improve your health.

The herb salvia crosses blood-brain barrier. It increases blood circulation. Salvia has both antiviral and antibiotic actions. Salvia is an anti-inflammatory. Salvia acts as sedative on the central nervous system. This herb might be useful in treating an undiagnosed virus that has damaged a brain. It could even help herpes 7 or herpes 8 infection that has not responded to other antiviral medications.

Brain trauma or head injury can be treated with salvia. The sedation effect of this herb and its antibiotic function improve the outcome for the brain trauma patient. The herb also protects the brain of the ischemia patient. This is due to the increase in circulation. It is important to begin the herb early in the medical treatment of brain trauma. It will work best if started within six weeks to six months of the initial injury.

Salvia's assistance for insomnia is likely due to the sedative affect of the drug. Salvia also can be used to treat cerebral thrombosis. The anti-inflammatory action and increase in circulation would allow the cerebral thrombosis to heal more quickly. Do not take salvia if you are taking anticoagulant or anti-platelet drugs. Do not take salvia if you are taking digoxin.

Passionflower is a sedative that can treat insomnia, anxiety, stress, depression, and neuralgia; it can increase circulation or lower blood pressure. Passionflower activates GABA receptors and is an analgesic and antispasmodic. It can prevent convulsions and can be taken as an anticonvulsant for epilepsy. It also can treat headaches and even has been used for treating delirium. It has antibacterial properties. Passionflower can be used as part of a strategy to treat nicotine addiction, alcoholism, and opiate withdrawal. Since addictions may become worse when people go extended periods of time without sleep, this herb can deal with both issues.

St. John's wort may be used to treat insomnia; it improves sleep quality and is a sedative. It has antiviral and antibacterial properties. It is an anxiolytic. It works in the brain affecting neurotransmitters by inhibiting the re-uptake of serotonin. It also has been used to treat anxiety, stress, depression, phobias, seasonal affective disorder, obsessive-compulsive disorder (OCD), and post-traumatic stress disorder (PTSD).

Acupuncture

Acupuncture is an ancient Chinese treatment for insomnia and depression. It works very quickly to solve the problem within a week to one month. Chronic insomnia usually will not be resolved within one week. It is often connected to drug abuse or alcoholism.

The main acupuncture tools are very thin needles, moxa, cupping, and electro-stimulation. Needles are inserted to points in the body. The acupuncture points, when needled, help balance the body's energy flow. Acupuncture can be used to treat stress and pain, generally or locally. Acupuncture is widely accepted for treatment of stress and has several mechanisms through which it addresses stress. It affects the cortex of the brain and the limbic system which provides a mechanism to treat stress, mood disorders, and addictions. Acupuncture can be used to treat stress without the side effects of drugs.

Acupuncture is effective in treating insomnia, narcolepsy, Parkinson's, Alzheimer's, autism, anxiety, insomnia, mood swings, depression, poor memory, PTSD, ischemia, ADD, ADHD, OCD, mania, hemiplegia, seizures, dizziness, epilepsy, stress, cognitive disorders, brain fog, and addictions. Acupuncture is clearly able to alter the levels of neurotransmitters in the brain. Scalp, auricular, body, and laser acupuncture will improve and heal stress. Acupuncture can be used along with Chinese herbal formulas for very quick stress relief.

Acupuncture points to help insomnia include Heart 7, Yin Tang, Shen Men, and An Mian.

Chinese Herbal Formulas to Use with Acupuncture

➢ An Mian Pian for quieting the spirit and quieting the mind

➢ Gui Pi Tang, which strengthens the energy and nourishes the heart

➢ Bao He Wan, which speeds the digestion time of food. It prevents food stagnation and harmonizes digestion for insomnia caused by late eating

➢ Zhu Sha An Shen Wan treats palpitations, heat, irritability, and insomnia

Bio-Mat

The Bio-Mat is a device that uses far infrared and amethyst crystals. The patient lies in the mat for twenty or thirty minutes and listens through earphones to sound and instructions. It seems like a meditation session, and it relaxes your body as the infrared speeds the elimination of toxins. This will reduce the toxic load on your liver, which is one way to reduce stress. It also ionizes your body with negative ions, which improves your body's ability to heal. This should normally be used about once or twice a week on the insomnia patient. The Bio-

Mat is a unique device that costs upwards of $2,500, depending on the size you choose. It is a patented device, and there is one manufacturer.

Aromatherapy

Aromatherapy is the controlled use of essential oil in treating insomnia, stress, and anxiety. It may be utilized by itself or as an adjunct therapy along with other mainstream and alternative medical treatments. It can be used in a vaporizer or in the top of a device that sits over a candle so that the heat interacts with the essential oil. Clinical research is currently being done in this field in England.

Try lavender, bergamot, rose, and freesia essential oils for treating insomnia, stress, and anxiety. Be very careful not to use the essential oils directly on the skin without diluting them into a base oil, such as grape seed oil. Essential oils can be expensive. They come in half-ounce and one ounce bottles. The essential oils will last longer if they are stored in dark blue or dark brown bottles.

Frankincense is a resin, and Traditional Chinese Medicine has used it as a Chinese herb for thousands of years. Frankincense incense significantly affected areas in brain areas known to be involved in emotions. It can be useful for insomnia, stress, and depression. Do not more than several drops of this essential oil at a time.

Exercise

Exercise can be used to treat or prevent insomnia. The exercise might be yoga, qi gong, walking, dancing, biking, golf, a gym work out, aerobics, ballet, swimming, tennis, or gardening. People with insomnia should be outside and exposed to sunlight at least thirty minutes per day.

Exercise reduces stress and should be done at least five days per week unless there is an injury that prevents it. If there is an injury, look for an exercise in yoga or qi gong that is performed while sitting in a chair. People who regularly engage in exercise or meditation show far less stress in their bodies. Their bodies age more slowly, and they experience less disease.

Binaural Beat, Hemi-Sync, or Metatone Therapy

Quantum Brain Healing uses binaural beat to treat insomnia, anxiety, depression, ADD, dementia, and addiction. The binaural beat developed by Dr. Robert Monroe of the Monroe Institute, is a sensory-information stimulus that changes the information sent to the reticular-thalamic activating system, which improves attention, focus, and level of awareness. It is a very unusual form of brain biofeedback that synchronizes brainwaves and can alter the brain-wave activity and balance between the left and right hemispheres. The Monroe Institute refers to this technology as Hemi-Sync. It reduces mental impairment and imbalances in the brain waves that need correction. This is achieved through extended exposure to the proper frequencies with a binaural beat. Binaural beats occur when different frequencies are delivered to the right and left hemispheres of the brain simultaneously.

Hemi-Sync signals contribute to a greater balance of activity of the right and left hemispheres and cortical and subcortical areas of the brain. Hemi-Sync can improve many brain diseases including dyslexia, Asperger's, Down's syndrome, autism, learning disabilities, developmentally disabled, ADHD, OCD, brain trauma, bipolar disorder, cerebral palsy, and seizure disorders, and improve cognitive function in children with borderline IQ. Children who are deaf, have a unilateral hearing loss, or absence of a brain structure such as the corpus callosum improve with Hemi-Sync.

Binaural beats are being researched by neurophysiologists to investigate their impact on hearing. Binaural beats are also studied for their ability to entrain brainwaves and their ability to be used for relaxation and health benefits. This is based upon the concept that brain disabilities and impairments are due to emotionally altered vibrations from your mind. Binaural beats alter the auric energy field of your brain in a negative way to change the type of brain wave or make the pattern of any type of brain wave irregular.

Dr. Monroe's binaural research has been taken to the next level in and further developed into Metatones.

Metatones can be used to treat insomnia, epilepsy, autism, addiction, learning disabilities, dementia, depression, anxiety, PTSD, Alzheimer's, dyslexia, ADHD, and closed head injury. Metatones is a vibratory medicine that is new and unconventional; this is not conventional music or sound therapy. Its founder considers it to be the next generation of sound therapy. It increases the rate of energy transfer in the brain. It is voice-activated, utilizing computer generated vocal permutations in a series of binaural beats to synchronize the brain waves. The audio programs escalate in vibration and resonance.

Biofeedback

Biofeedback may be used for psychological and stress problems. Biofeedback works directly on the brain. The brain is the computer for the body that drives most of its activities. Biofeedback can also be used to treat addiction issues. Many people suffer from insomnia, chronic headaches, migraines, sexual dysfunction, nervous stomach, essential hypertension, repetitive strain injury (RSI), brain fog, anger management issues, tics, and neuropathy. Many times, multiple therapies are needed, and this is a good tool. Biofeedback may be better for some people who have diseases that are rooted in stress.

Chronic stress can cause some very serious problems. Chronic stress often leads to over-activation of the sympathetic nervous system, which is responsible for actions that are uncontrollable by conscious thought, like blood pressure, hormones, increases in heart rate, and the constriction of blood vessels. The body works to achieve a balanced state, and many times it is unable to do so. This causes stress-related disease. The immune system fails under excessive, long-term chronic stress, and symptoms and diseases surface.

Biofeedback machines can help people manage their bodies' reactions to reduce stress-related diseases. Insomnia caused by stress or anxiety can be resolved or improved. High blood pressure can be managed for some people with biofeedback. ADD, ADHD, anxiety, headaches, and migraines related to elevated blood pressure can fade. Addictions will be more easily dealt with and treated. Low-back pain can be treated with biofeedback. Teeth grinding and TMJ can improve with this therapy. It has also been used for seizure disorders and epilepsy of unknown origin. This may be used as a preventative to avoid or delay the onset of an autoimmune disease. It will take several sessions, and each session generally lasts about one hour. The sessions are moderately priced.

Qi Gong

Qi gong is an ancient type of Chinese energy work that can transform anyone's health. It increases activity in the pre-frontal cortex and amygdala. It can heal anxiety and sleep disorders. It increases brain relaxation, reduces stress, and treats mild to moderate depression. Qi gong can improve oxygen levels. This improves positive thoughts and is very helpful for people in recovery from serious disease, like cancer, ischemia, MS, or stroke.

This is an energy form that has many benefits similar to tai chi, Therapeutic Touch, and Reiki. Qi gong influences electromagnetic energy throughout the body. It can change electrical activity in the body, balance blood flow, and cellular water balance. This type of energy work is a slow and controlled movement of the body and its qi. The correct movement by the body can improve its energy. Long-term qi gong will help improve energy levels, improve sleep, and balance hormones and neurotransmitters. It can be done in a group setting or by yourself.

A qi gong device is available that moves your legs and feet for you. This will help those who do not have the ability to stand, such as people with vertigo, Parkinson's, or significant disabilities. It sells for about $140 and can be ordered online. There is also a hand-held device that delivers energy, which is supposed to be similar to that of qi gong. I have not tested that particular device and can offer only the thought that it might be better than nothing.

Qi gong has many movements, and some may be difficult to recall. The use of a DVD can help the qi gong practice of a novice. The medical impact of qi gong includes increasing brain circulation, lowering or increasing blood pressure levels toward a moderate level, and balancing endocrine gland function. Qi gong improves hormone and neurotransmitter levels. It helps you sleep better. It reduces hypertension and helps manage asthma. This form of ancient Chinese energy work decreases the occurrence of strokes and improves your sex life. It is anti-aging and increases your immune function. People live longer after including a long-term qi gong practice in their lives.

Qi gong may be adapted to a chair with arm and upper body movements in order to stimulate and heal the body. It can even be done in a hospital bed. Energy work can reduce the cost of health care throughout the world. The person without depression or anxiety is less prone to disease because his immune system is functioning at a higher level.

Yoga

There are several yoga poses that are wonderful for helping balance the body to treat insomnia. These poses include Downward Facing Dog, Cat Pose, Child Pose, Easy Pose, Head to Knee Pose, Corpse Pose, and Fire Log Pose. Yoga is a great way to increase circulation, improve flexibility, reduce stress, balance hormone function, restore proper sleep cycles, and improve energy flow. Your yoga practice balances neurotransmitters and hormones to relax your body and restore normal sleep patterns. Yoga postures can be done at home on the floor to help you sleep during times of high stress. Yoga postures may be practiced for ten minutes before bedtime to help you fall asleep.

Power yoga is aerobic in nature and will burn more calories and improve circulation more quickly. It requires that the participant be healthy. A yoga posture, or asana, may be repeated quickly several times. There are standing and floor postures. Power yoga classes usually last one hour. This active aerobic yoga class, done on a regular basis, will help establish regular sleep patterns. Try to do power yoga before the evening in order to get best results, relative to insomnia problems.

Hatha yoga increases balance, flexibility, and fitness at a gentle pace suitable for almost everyone. People of ages and levels of fitness can do this yoga. It is very important to discuss all health problems with the yoga instructor prior to class so you can be guided in which postures need to be avoided for specific health concerns.

Bikram yoga, or hot yoga, is a great way to detoxify, increase flexibility, and increase metabolism. This practice involves performing yoga postures for ninety minutes in a heated room. The first half of the session involves standing postures, while the second half of the class is floor postures. Because muscles are warm, most people are able to increase flexibility at a faster rate. It is important to take water with you to class. Do not push yourself in this class until you are experienced in how the heat will affect you. Do not do Bikram yoga every day, as it can result in electrolyte imbalances. If you are feeling dizzy after class, replenish your electrolytes with a supplement.

MANIA

Quantum Brain Healing treats mania as one its more challenging and difficult diseases. Early diagnosis is key. Mania patients need medical intervention early for a good outcome. Mania is a mood disorder that includes extreme elevated mood, rapid speech, psychosis, poor judgment, restlessness, hallucinations, excess gambling, reckless sex, excess spending, excess computer gaming, extreme disregard for the feelings of others, increased selfishness, grandiose schemes, extreme insomnia, high energy, and abnormal thought patterns. Crime may be an element for some patients with mania, as there is an element of belief that one cannot get caught or can do no wrong.

Many factors can trigger mania, including stress, failure, food allergies, allergic reactions to over-the-counter and prescription drugs, excess caffeine, heavy-metals poisoning, environmental poisoning, trauma, sexual or physical abuse, and extreme emotional abuse. Children raised without parents experience this disease more frequently.

People with mania should avoid strobe lights, black lights, psychedelic rock music, continuous extremely loud noise, long-term overwork, and excess visual stimulation, like extreme violence, pornography, excess computer gaming, or computer work. There is a high degree of co-morbidity of mood disorders with OCD, ADD, alcoholism, drug addiction, and sexual addiction. Good nutrition is very important in managing any mood disorder. A peaceful home environment and avoiding stress are very important in managing mania.

Patients need to be aware of the symptoms that occur prior to an event of mania so that it can be avoided or managed quickly. The symptoms include insomnia, giddiness, very bad decisions, eating pattern changes, appetite increase, appetite decrease, trouble concentrating, listlessness, or tiredness.

Quantum Brain Healing focuses on diagnosing the problem and looking at issues like exposure to poisons and toxins. Mania may be a side effect of an overdose of a medicine; it is frequently a side effect of extreme drug abuse.

The toxins in cigarettes may cause or contribute to mania. In young children, it is important to consider allergic reactions or food allergies when mania is diagnosed. Many children have very extreme allergies that may have been incorrectly diagnosed as ADHD, mania, or other mood disorders. Mania and hypomania may be associated with creativity and artistic talent. The risk of having this disease increases when a close family member has been diagnosed.

Mania can be associated with manic depression or bipolar disorder, but it can also be caused by drugs, such as stimulants like cocaine. St. John's wort, Rhodiola rosea, horny goat weed, ginseng, and SAM-e supplementation need to be closely monitored to avoid increasing the magnitude of the mania. Any stimulating supplement should be avoided. These supplements can also be triggers for bipolar patients, turning depression into mania. Electro-convulsive therapy can trigger suicide in patients with mania. Electro-cranial stimulation could also result in overstimulation and result in mania for a person having the disease.

Excessive thyroid levels may create some symptoms that resemble mania or hypomania, such as insomnia, hyperactivity, or increased energy. It is important for mood disorder patients to have their vitamin, mineral, and hormone levels tested, as many mood disorders are vitamin, mineral, or hormone imbalances that are undiagnosed. Mood disorders may produce elevated daily requirements of certain vitamins or minerals. Nutritional supplementation can resolve mood disorders or reduce mania events for some patients.

Vitamins

Treating diseases with Orthomolecular Medicine usually requires higher levels of a substance than are found in most vitamin supplements or in foods. Diseases frequently increase the level of a vitamin or mineral needed in the body to maintain good health. The RDA of vitamins and minerals is insufficient for most people with illness, and their metabolism may have altered. This may result is a lower level of bio-availability of their nutrients.

Brain Healing uses vitamin B12 to heal mania if the disease is caused by a vitamin B12 deficiency. B12 is involved in DNA synthesis and fatty acid synthesis, and it helps break down carbohydrates and covert them into energy. It is used by the body to help make several amino acids, including SAM-e. These amino acids are found to change brain chemistry and neurotransmitter levels. The neurotransmitters affected by vitamin B12 directly are involved in learning skills and memory. Vitamin B12 is found in beef, caviar, chicken, cheese, eggs, fish, lamb, liver, milk, octopus, and shellfish. A sublingual form of this vitamin is available. A multivitamin product should also be taken with this supplement so that the other B vitamins do not become deficient.

Symptoms of vitamin B12 deficiency include mania, fatigue, brain fog, delusion, poor memory, neurological problems, poor concentration, depression, psychosis, irritability, forgetfulness, and increased sleep requirements. These symptoms may also be indicative of other vitamin or mineral deficiencies. Any of the above conditions may be treated with B12 if a deficiency exists. Many people have multiple vitamin deficiencies, and all deficiencies must be treated for the patient to heal.

Quantum Orthomolecular Medicine uses higher amounts of vitamin B12 than would be found in multivitamin product or normal diet. Many brain diseases may require these higher levels of vitamin B12 in order for healing to occur. Diseases improved by taking vitamin B12 include Alzheimer's disease, dementia, depression, long-term memory loss, and impaired ability to convert short-term memory into long-term memory. The brain fog symptom associated with chronic fatigue syndrome can be improved with increased doses of B12. It is always worth noting that digestive problems may be the root of vitamin deficiencies. A digestive enzyme may allow you to better absorb most of your vitamins.

Melatonin is a hormone precursor and may be used in doses up to 3 mg per day and taken at night, thirty minutes prior to bedtime. This will help balance the brain and your circadian rhythm cycle. It should improve your sleep. Melatonin will cross the blood-brain barrier and increase brain circulation. It increases the production of neurotransmitters and balances the brain. It strengthens the immune system. The enhanced immune system is due to the improvement in hormone and neurotransmitter regulation.

Vitamin C can be taken in doses from 1 to 3 grams per day as an antioxidant and detoxification agent. It will help your body fight stress and support your immune system.

Coenzyme Q10 or CoQ10 is a ubiquinone and is a cofactor in energy production. This coenzyme is used in energy production by the mitochondria. CoQ10 affects many neurological functions. It is best taken with food that contains some type of lipid or fat. Take this with some type of fat or oil or foods that contain fat or oil, such as walnuts, almonds, salmon, a small amount of butter on a vegetable, cold-press extra virgin olive oil, walnut oil, almond oil, sesame oil, or pine nuts.

CoQ10 should be taken in large amounts for neuropathy and at the same time as alpha lipoic acid is taken with pure water. CoQ10 should be taken for several years to see the full effect and obtain all its benefits. It is active in the central cortex of the brain. It enhances immune function, is an antioxidant, and reduces migraine headaches. It protects brain cells and protects pancreatic beta cells from type 2 diabetes. It crosses the blood-brain barrier. It will help increase energy production by the cells, reduce fatigue, and protect against memory loss. It can help neuropathy and brain diseases like ALS.

Quantum Brain Healing may treat mania with lithium orotate, a trace mineral salt found in RNA and DNA that helps balance neurotransmitter levels and stimulates the repair of damaged nerve tissue. This mineral salt can travel inside the brain and stabilize many of the chemical activities of the neurons or brain cells. It protects brain cells in the hippocampus, striatum, and frontal cortex of the brain. It helps support neural plasticity, reduces mental stress, and stimulates the growth of new neurons.

Use lithium orotate in therapeutic doses for a least one year before discontinuing. If symptoms return, continue to take this mineral salt. Lithium orotate can help stabilize the patient with schizophrenia when he or she is not taking drugs, narcotics, alcohol, or nicotine. It is very effective for moderate to severe depression that does not respond to drugs. The moderately depressed patient may also need to add therapeutic doses of amino acids. The levels of supplements will have to be monitored very closely - it is difficult to predict the exact amounts needed of lithium orotate and how it will react with other medicines or nutritional supplements. Bipolar disorder can also be treated with lithium orotate.

Alpha lipoic acid should be taken in fairly large amounts, up to 400 mg per day, by patients experiencing mania. This dosage should be weight-adjusted for teenagers. The dosage of 400 mg per day would be for a weight of 150 pounds.

Diet

Diet and nutrition can help manage and treat mania. The challenge is to determine which Quantum Brain Healing recommendation works the best for the patient. The elimination diet, rotation diet, ketogenic diet, and GARD work well. The rotation diet involves rotating the foods in your diet to eat each food no more than once during any given four-day period. Keep foods local and organic. Drink organic caffeine-free teas and low-sugar vegetable and fruit juices.

The elimination diet involves the elimination of foods from your diet and re-introduction of the food item after it has been removed for at least one month. Bring back one food at a time so that you can identify the problem food. The key is to stop or greatly eliminate the stimulating foods and substances in your diet. Restricting diet to a healthy, balanced diet with five small meals per day to manage glucose levels helps improve mania.

People with mania need to limit sugar, carbonated beverages, alcohol, tobacco, caffeine, refined foods, food additives, artificial sweeteners, chocolate, recreational drugs, over-the-counter drugs, preservatives, and food dyes. They should include organic and local fruits and vegetables, pure fresh water, adequate high-quality protein, untested raw nuts, extra virgin olive oil, organic caffeine-free herbal teas, salmon, mackerel, cod, sardines, and Swiss method decaffeinated coffee where coffee is decaffeinated with water. Avoid foods that have a high level of vanadium.

Ketogenic Diet

The ketogenic diet is a high-fat, low-carbohydrate diet with a moderate to high amount of protein. It can be used to help mania, but it is not an overnight fix. The diet increases the energy production in the hippocampus, helps the brain to become more resistant to reduced glucose levels, and increases the brain's ability to handle metabolism changes.

This diet is heavily supplemented with vitamins and minerals. It should be done under the care of a registered dietician or physician. Fluids are restricted, so that electrolytes do not get out of balance. This is a difficult diet with few food choices, and it can moderate electrical activity in the brain if used more than one to two years. The ketogenic diet produces an effect similar to starvation and forces the body to burn fat instead of carbohydrates. Calories are strictly controlled so that weight is not lost or gained during the diet. Regular growth and repair of the body continues.

When glucose is not sufficient, the body burns fat. The fat is not completely burned and ketones are formed. The high level of ketones seems to reduce or eliminate seizures in many people. This diet seems to alter the seizure threshold with the elevation of ketone levels. In 1998, Johns Hopkins Medical School released a study on the ketogenic diet, showing the diet significantly helped eliminate the seizure activity in approximately one-third of the patients studied. Other patients showed reduced seizure activity. The mechanism of this diet is to alter glucose metabolism and increase energy production and stabilize the brain. These actions and others make this diet worth trying for mania. Side effects of the ketogenic diet include dehydration, kidney stones, constipation, vomiting, increased cholesterol, lower growth rate, behavior changes, and mood changes.

Glutamate-Aspartate Restricted Diet (GARD)

The GARD is a type of elimination diet developed to treat epilepsy in animals; it identifies foods and ingredients that should be avoided, including the following:

- gluten; commonly derived from wheat and grains
- casein; protein found in cow's milk (and most dairy products)
- soy
- corn, including corn syrup and corn derivative products
- MSG (monosodium glutamate); this a very common food ingredient in processed foods, even though it is rarely clearly labeled as such
- aspartame; commonly used as a sugar substitute
- glutamate; found in high concentrations in most beans/legumes
- hydrogenated oils

The GARD is a glutamate-aspartate restricted diet due to the limitation of these two nonessential, neurostimulating amino acids that are also the parent compounds of MSG and aspartame (NutraSweet). Aspartame is a neurotoxin that has been connected with brain cancer in Italy. Glutamate and aspartate are excitotoxins. They are able to trigger seizures and cause neurodegenerative diseases in some patients. The GARD is also referred to as the "gut absorption recovery diet" due to its removal of gluten, dairy, soy, and corn. These foods may induce damage to the intestinal villi, resulting in celiac disease and food intolerance.

There is little or no published clinical research for the GARD. If effective, this diet needs to be adopted as a permanent lifestyle change. GARD allows high-glycemic and high-carbohydrates foods. Diabetics, hypoglycemics, or anyone who has a sensitivity to dietary sugars should try the GARD only under the strict supervision of their doctor. This diet may help many people that suffer with food allergies.

The following are other nutritional options for mania:

- Single dose of 1 to 6 grams vitamin C
- Melatonin; as a sleep aid
- Lecithin supplement
- Omega-3 fatty acids
- Flaxseed oil
- Black cohosh; acts as a nervous system depressant, sedative, anti-inflammatory
- Sarsaparilla;a nervous system depressant, sedative, and anti-anxiolitic
- White Pumpkin (Ayurvedic medicine)
- Skullcap
- Valerian

Intravenous Nutritional Therapy or the Myers Cocktail

The Myers Cocktail is an intravenous therapy consisting of mixing vitamins, minerals, amino acids, and other nutrients. It can be very useful in treating autoimmune diseases, chronic illness, viral infections, or digestive problems where oral nutrients are not being absorbed. When nutrients are given intravenously, your digestive system is bypassed and a much higher level of nutrition can be delivered directly to your cells via the bloodstream. Dr. John Myers was the first doctor to develop an intravenous nutrient therapy that obtained positive clinical results for a variety of medical conditions. Be very careful to get the full amount of the vitamins in the IV. Some doctors offices are putting fewer vitamins into the IV bag to save money. Ask specific questions the amount levels of the vitamins and minerals.

Mania can occur for many reasons, but mineral imbalances are prevalent in many cases of mania. The ratio of minerals to one another may be off or simply deficient to extreme levels. Heavy metals are often found in brain tissue of people suffering from mania. IV therapy is wonderful after detoxification of heavy metals with oral chelators.

Treating mania requires an extra large IV therapy lasting about two and one-half hours. Reversing mineral imbalances in a case of mania will require about fourteen to thirty IV treatments. Any drug addiction issues must also be treated. Tobacco products must be avoided to avoid a relapse of mania symptoms. Any product high in toxins should be eliminated. This can include shampoo, make-up, dry cleaning chemicals in clothing, chemicals in high refined foods, car cleaning chemicals, and chemicals in coffee and alcohol. Deficient immune systems can rebound after three sessions of the Myers Cocktail.

The Myers Cocktail improves almost all digestive symptoms including bloating, diarrhea, food allergies, irritable bowel syndrome, colitis, ulcers, black mold exposure, environmental allergies, cancer, and Crohn's disease. The Myers Cocktail intravenous therapy improves the body's ability to make energy and increases cellular function. It also speeds the cells ability to remove cellular waste. Your cells produce higher levels of ATP. If your arm begins to hurt or get sore after the IV begins, ask the nurse to slow the rate of the IV drip. The beneficial effect is usually fast, but extremely ill people will require several IV treatments to feel better.

The Myers Cocktail IV therapy may be helpful for chronic or acute conditions, including digestive problems, mental fatigue, PTSD, fatigue, fibromyalgia, depression, bacterial or viral infection, asthma, cardiac pain, congestive heart failure, palpitations, migraine headaches, cardiovascular disease, respiratory problems, seasonal allergies, hives, hyperthyroidism, and muscle spasms due to nutritional deficiency.

NAET

NAET can be used to treat and improve mania. Mania may be an acute problem if it is due to heavy-metals or pesticide poisoning. Acute mania may respond quickly to NAET treatment. Chronic mania is quite difficult to treat; it is possible to improve rather than cure this problem. This is especially true if this is an inherited illness. Most diseases are impacted by environmental or food allergies. Mania patients should be treated for allergens. This will help the immune system improve and therefore improve the patient's prognosis. It will not work on all people. NAET will require about two treatments per week; treatments last approximately thirty-five to forty-five minutes over a period of approximately one year. The severity of the case and the age of the patient will determine the number of sessions required.

Nambudripad's Allergy Elimination Technique (NAET) is a technique to eliminate allergies of all types and levels using a blend of medical therapies taken from acupuncture or acupressure, allopathy, chiropractic, nutrition, and kinesiology. It can be noninvasive when acupressure is utilized. It is pain-free, but there may be the presentation of allergic symptoms during the twenty-five hour period following the treatment. The patient needs to be rested, hydrated, and not hungry for an optimal treatment. There is usually an avoidance period of twenty-five hours after the treatment, where specific items need to be avoided. These items or foods will be identified for the patient at the time of treatment.

One allergen is treated at a time. If you are not severely immune deficient, you may need just one treatment to desensitize one allergen. Mania patients often have overactive immune systems. Look for environmental allergies, drug exposure, chemicals, and electro-magnetic pollution. Additional symptoms such as depression, anxiety, insomnia, memory loss, and alcoholism will require additional attention and treatment. A person with mild to moderate allergies may need fifteen to twenty office visits to desensitize fifteen to twenty food and environmental allergens. Basic essential nutrients are treated and cleared during the first few visits.

It is important to diagnose and treat the primary allergens that negatively affect the body's ability to maintain health. The longer an allergy goes untreated, the more inflammation occurs. Ordinary items that are not allergens will cause a reaction in a body that is in a state of high inflammation. Extremely ill people with many allergies may require an extended period to get well, but there should be some improvement shown after the initial fifteen to twenty treatments. Acute situations, such as food poisoning, can respond within two hours.

The website to locate a trained NAET practitioner anywhere in the world is www.NAET.com. If you are not satisfied with the initial treatment, seek another NAET doctor for the follow-up treatments. It is important to get the right doctor and follow your treatment plan.

Heavy-Metals Poisoning

Heavy-metals poisoning creates many health problems today. Toxin exposure may be encountered in bad water, food, air, the workplace, reclaimed soil, toxic waste site, refuse disposal sites, and vaccines. Conditions and diseases related to heavy-metals poisoning may include impaired cognitive skills, insomnia, depression, anxiety, stress, ADHD, obsessive-compulsive disorder (OCD), impaired digestion, neuropathy, colitis, delirium, hallucination, fatigue and chronic fatigue, impaired concentration, brain fog, numbness, hair loss, impaired liver function, cancer, weakness, learning disabilities, dementia, and stupor. Symptoms and diseases vary for different heavy metals.

Mercury poisoning can cause social withdrawal or interaction problems, depression, mood disorders, aggressive behavior, OCD, autism, insomnia, delirium, hallucinations, fatigue and chronic fatigue, eating disorders, suicidal threats, ADHD, weakness, speech problems, colitis, difficulty walking, temper tantrums, hearing loss, convulsions, seizures, birth defects, spontaneous abortion, motor problems, rashes, skin problems, nausea, vomiting, diarrhea, stomach cramps, allergies, asthma, and neurological problems.

Aluminum poisoning can cause Alzheimer's, fatigue and chronic fatigue, weakness, dementia, skin problems, rashes, motor disturbances, neurological problems, allergies, asthma, infertility issues, and respiratory diseases.

Lead poisoning can cause memory problems, concentration difficulty, depression, mood swings, irritability, insomnia, sleep disturbance, anxiety, eating disorders, ADHD, mental retardation, impaired intelligence, birth defects, spontaneous abortion, neurological problems, convulsions, seizures, headaches, muscle pain, hypertension, cardiac problems, and suppressed immune function.

The skin is a major organ through which the body detoxifies. Our body also filters toxins from the blood system (detoxification) through the liver, kidneys, gallbladder, and the lymphatic system. It is important to detoxify these systems by drinking plenty of pure water. There are several ways to reduce the heavy-metals load on the body, including diet, nutritional supplements, intravenous chelation therapy, far infrared sauna, foot ionizing detoxification, hot yoga, and any exercise that produces sweat.

IV chelation therapy is administered in a doctor's office usually over several hours. It involves injecting ethylenediaminetetraacetic acid (EDTA) into the bloodstream to remove heavy metals, chemical toxins, mineral deposits, and fatty plaques. EDTA is a synthetic amino acid chelating agent for most metals other than mercury. DMSA and DMPS are chemicals used intravenously to chelate mercury, but are not approved by the FDA. The nutritional supplements include cilantro, barley, wheatgrass, alfalfa, kelp, alpha lipoic acid, L-cysteine, methionine, vitamin C, garlic, MSM, and pectin.

Biofeedback

Biofeedback may be used for psychological and stress problems. It can also be used to treat addiction issues. Many people suffer from chronic headaches, migraines, sexual dysfunction, migraines, mania, nervous stomach, sex addictions, compulsive shopping addictions, MS, Huntington's disease, stress, trichotillomania, IQ enhancement, essential hypertension, repetitive strain injury (RSI), brain fog, anger management issues, tics, and neuropathy. Many times, multiple therapies are needed, and this is a good tool. Biofeedback may be better for some people who have diseases that are rooted in stress.

Mania is not cured with biofeedback. This is a stress management tool for the high stress level of the disease. Chronic stress can cause some very serious problems. Chronic stress often leads to over-activation of the sympathetic nervous system, which is responsible for our actions that are uncontrolled by conscious thought, like blood pressure, hormones, increases in heart rate, or the constriction of blood vessels. The body works to achieve a balanced state, and many times it has been unable to do so. This causes stress related disease. The immune system fails under excessive long-term chronic stress, and symptoms and diseases surface.

Biofeedback machines can help people manage their bodies' reactions to reduce stress related diseases. Insomnia caused by stress or anxiety can be resolved or improved. High blood pressure can be managed for some people with biofeedback. ADD, ADHD, anxiety, headaches, and migraines related to elevated blood pressure can fade. Addictions will be more easily dealt with and treated. Low-back pain can be treated with biofeedback. Teeth grinding and TMJ can improve with this therapy. It has also been used for seizure disorders and epilepsy of unknown origin. This may be used as a preventative to avoid or delay the onset of an autoimmune disease. It will take several sessions, and each session generally lasts about one hour. The sessions are moderately priced.

Alternative Therapies for Mania

- Acupuncture
- Scalp acupuncture
- Auricular acupuncture
- Orthomolecular therapy
- Yoga
- Tai chi
- Qi gong
- Prayer
- Meditation
- Cognitive behavioral therapy
- Playing a musical instrument
- Cranial sacral therapy
- Music therapy
- Bach Flower Remedies
- Exercise that is not overstimulating, such as walking, gardening, biking, playing

golf, bowling, fishing, and flying a kite; and avoidance of extreme sports, such as downhill skiing, car racing or motorcycle racing

- ➤ Eight to nine hours sleep each night
- ➤ Daily light exposure for no more than one hour
- ➤ Creation of health care and personal support networks
- ➤ Focus on self-acceptance
- ➤ Introducing joy on a daily basis into your life
- ➤ Color therapy
- ➤ EMDR (eye movement desensitization and reprocessing)
- ➤ Medical marijuana or cannabinoids

Herbs

Skullcap may be used to treat brain disease including epilepsy, ADD, headaches, neuralgia, insomnia, hysteria, anxiety, delirium, and convulsions. Skullcap can be used in addiction disorders for symptoms like withdrawal from barbiturates, alcohol, and tranquilizers. This Quantum Brain herb should be used in an overall treatment plan for those suffering from addictions. Preventing brain disease and protecting the brain is an important step in your anti-aging program. It is possible to remove up to twenty biological years from your brain with alternative therapies and herbal medicine. This allows the prevention and delayed onset of many brain diseases. You can work longer and perform complex tasks with ease. This herb can help calm the overstimulated brain and reduce mania symptoms when taken in small doses three to five times per day for up to 18 days.

Lemon balm is used in Quantum Brain Healing to treat mania and other primary brain disease or secondary brain disease symptoms. Lemon balm is a sedative and antioxidant. It can be used to treat stress and anxiety. Its sedative effect can benefit nervous exhaustion. Lemon balm has strong medical properties and mildness. It is an antiviral and antibiotic agent. It can act as an antidepressant for mild depression. Lemon balm acts on the hippocampus area of the brain and functions as an antispasmodic. Lemon balm can help clear the brain for enhanced learning for those with a brain disease. This herb acts on the brain in many ways to reduce signs of aging. Aging of the brain may be accelerated by bacterial and viral infections that go undiagnosed and untreated. Any herb that has antibiotic and antiviral actions may be taken on a regular basis to prevent infection or accelerated aging.

Catuaba is a South American herb that has many medical properties, including the ability to act as an antibiotic and antiviral. It also is an adaptogen and can sedate or stimulate the brain and central nervous system as needed. It is an antioxidant and may be an amino anti-aging

164

herb for the brain. Catuaba is an analgesic for the brain and can calm the brain when over-stimulation as occurred. Serious infection causes brain symptoms that are similar to over-stimulation due to the nature of heat in the brain. Mania is one of the primary diseases that can fall into the over-stimulation category. Quantum Brain Healing uses several adaptogens for brain support during substance withdrawal. This herb should be tried for a short time, and if there is no improvement, discontinue after two weeks.

Chinese Herbal Formulas

> **Bu Nao Wan**, Supplement the Brain Pills or Clear Mind from Kan

Traditional Chinese Medicine (TCM) therapeutic effects include tonifying heart yin, blood, and liver blood, transforming heart phlegm, calming the shen, nourishing the brain, strengthening the kidneys, and eliminating liver wind. Clear Mind is a Chinese herbal formula used to treat an overactive mind, mania, OCD, depression, anxiety, mental agitation, restlessness, fatigue, and insomnia and enhance concentration or memory.

> **Gun Tan Wan**, Vaporize Phlegm Pill or Chasing Away Phlegm Pill

TCM therapeutic effects include treating heat, phlegm-heat and phlegm-fire. Vaporize Phlegm Pill is a Chinese herbal formula used to treat acute mania, anxiety, neurosis, dizziness, hysteria, nervous breakdown, heart palpitations, episodic mania, schizophrenia, bipolar disorder, tinnitus, acute bronchitis, agitated dreams, bizarre dreams, and coma.

> **Bu Zhong Yi Qi Wan** or Supplement the Center and Boost the Qi Decoction

TCM therapeutic effects include tonifying qi, tonifying spleen qi, and lifting yang. Supplement the Center and Boost the Qi Decoction is a Chinese herbal formula used to treat anxiety, mania, various phobias, cerebral arteriosclerosis, dizziness, and stress.

> **Di Dang Tang** or Resistance Decoction

TCM therapeutic effects include treating blood stasis and draining heat downward. Resistance Decoction is a Chinese herbal formula used to treat severe or extreme mania.

> **Ding Xian Wan**, Stopping Epilepsy Pill; Arrest Seizures Pill; Gastrodia and Succinum Pill

TCM therapeutic effects include treating phlegm, wind, liver-wind, and opening the orifices. Arrest Seizures Pill is a Chinese herbal formula used to treat acute mania, dementia, nervous breakdown, bipolar disorder, clonic convulsion, infantile epilepsy, piercing scream, recurrent dizziness, alcohol and drug withdrawal, and dementia.

➤ **Huang Lian Jie Du Pian** or Coptis Relieve Toxicity

TCM therapeutic effects include treating heat from all three burners, blood heat, toxic heat, fire, damp heat, liver heat, and heart heat. Coptis Relieving Toxicity is a Chinese herbal formula used to treat mania, insomnia, bad breath, bleeding, delirium, palpitations, blood in stools or urine, incoherent speech, anxiety, emotional instability, and dysentery.

➤ **Sheng Tie Luo Yin** or Iron Filings Decoction

TCM therapeutic effects include treating phlegm, phlegm-fire, calming the heart, and calming the mind. Iron Filings Decoction is a Chinese herbal formula used to treat bad temper, extreme emotional instability, insomnia, irritability, mania, restlessness, aggressiveness, and screaming.

➤ **Tao He Cheng Qi Tang** or Peach Pit Decoction to Order the Qi

TCM therapeutic effects include treating blood stasis, blood accumulation, and blood heat in the lower Jiao. Peach Pit Decoction to Order the Qi is a Chinese herbal formula used to treat acute mania, irritability, restlessness, acute lower abdominal pain, delirium, dysmenorrhea, endometriosis, intestinal obstruction, and irregular menstruation.

Acupuncture

Acupuncture is an ancient Chinese treatment to treat mania. It is usually combined with herbs. It is a holistic approach in treating and preventing disease. The main acupuncture tools are very thin needles, moxibustion, cupping, and electro-stimulation. Needles are inserted to points in the body. It modulates the limbic system, which provides a mechanism to treat mood disorders and addictions. Acupuncture can be used to treat many mood disorders and mental imbalances with an efficacy equal to pharmacology, without the side effects of drugs.

Acupuncture is effective in treating mania and addictions. Mania may arise from a parasite infection that passes the blood-brain barrier and gets into the brain. It may also be the result of bacterial and viral infections. Fungal infections may cause a symptom that resembles mania. Acupuncture is very good at calming the brain. Mania has extreme reactions, and acupuncture balances the body and brain to bring it into homeostasis. These problems can all be dramatically improved with acupuncture. The success of acupuncture arises from several factors, including patient compliance, diet, exercise, medical history, and practitioner expertise.

Auricular acupuncture is often used to treat mania. The auricular points used for mania include shen men, heart 1, subcortex, brain, brain stem, cortex, and zero point. Several sessions will be required, and each session will take from thirty to forty-five minutes. Mourant acupuncture adds silver needles to this treatment, along with a sound meditation of violin or chanting from a monastery.

Scalp acupuncture treatments can also be used. The ear or the scalp may be successful for the treatment of mania. Body points also can be used and include amnian, stomach 41, heart 7, heart 9, small intestine 3, heart 9, lung 11, urinary bladder 8, urinary bladder 15, urinary bladder 62, urinary bladder 63, urinary bladder 65, urinary bladder 66, pericardium 7, du 18, du 19, du 20, ren 1, and ren 14.

Yoga

Yoga is a great way to increase circulation, improve flexibility, reduce stress, balance hormone function, restore proper sleep cycles, and improve energy flow. There are many types of yoga that offer different health benefits.

Power yoga is aerobic in nature and will burn more calories and improve circulation more quickly. It requires that the participant be healthy. A yoga posture, or asana, may be repeated quickly several times. There are standing and floor postures. Power yoga classes usually last one hour. This class would be very good for mania. The key to yoga is stopping when you are overtaxed.

Hatha yoga increases balance, flexibility, and fitness at a gentle pace suitable for almost everyone. People of ages and levels of fitness can do this yoga. It is very important to discuss all health problems with the yoga instructor prior to class so you can be guided in which postures you need to avoid for specific health concerns.

Bikram yoga, or hot yoga, is a great way to detoxify, increase flexibility, and increase metabolism. This practice involves performing yoga postures for ninety minutes in a heated room. The first half of the session involves standing postures, while the second half of the class is floor postures. Because your muscles are warm, most people are able to increase flexibility at a faster rate. It is important to take water with you to class. Do not push yourself in this class until you are experienced in how the heat will affect you. Do not do this yoga every day, as it can result in electrolyte imbalances. If you are feeling dizzy after class, replenish your electrolytes with a supplement.

If you have arthritis or other motion-limiting issues, herbs may improve your yoga practice and take it to the next level. Herbs can increase flexibility, promote circulation, and stimulate the movement of energy. Herbs can aid in the proper performance of postures by improving circulation, joint function, balance, and coordination. They may be referred to as antirheumatic or anti-arthritic agents.

-

Yoga is an amazing tool for athletic people for interrupting chronic pain. Professional athletes often have success in using Bikram yoga to replace strong pain medications to solve chronic pain after the muscle or ligament tears have healed.

Several yoga poses can help balance the body to treat mania. The entire yoga series can be used for improving yoga. The Child Pose can be done for five to seven minutes to calm reduce mania.

Eye Movement Desensitization and Reprocessing (EMDR)

EMDR may have use in mania in an indirect manner. It helps treat emotional issues of all types, including childhood trauma, automobile accidents, assault, natural disasters, sexual assault, personal failures, divorce, panic attacks, phobias, sexual addiction, computer or Nintendo addiction, and combat trauma. This is can be very effective for a person who has been gang-raped or assaulted by a gang or in a riot. EMDR may significantly help mania that has been triggered by an event rather than genetics. It could be massive stress tied to a nuclear meltdown at a power plant, radiation, earthquake, hurricane, tsunami, tornado, or mountain slide. The concept is a life-shaping event.

The doctor must initially analyze the patient's current situations that trigger unemotional disturbance and evaluate past traumatic events to determine if the patient currently has the needed coping skills to prevent a similar circumstance from arising. If the patient has the skills, then the doctor may move forward.

A specific memory or event is identified and processed using EMDR procedures. The patient identifies the most specific image related to the memory and whatever negative feelings of self-worth are tied to this event. This is processed along with the sensations and feelings of the patient that are tied to this event. These feelings may include fear, nausea, headaches, crying, trauma, and inadequacy. The patient is given a positive image and belief to substitute for the problematic feeling or event. The intensity of the negative emotions should diminish during this treatment, and a positive emotion will root the patient.

The doctor helps the patient focus on the event and negative feeling while body sensations are created. The patient moves his eyes rapidly and follows the doctor's fingers as they move for approximately thirty to sixty seconds. The eye movements are used by all doctors, but some doctors may add auditory sounds and tapping, similar to Emotional Freedom Technique

(EFT). The doctor asks the patient to describe the sensations that are being processed. This therapy can work wonders for people experiencing massive amounts of fear, hysteria, mania, anger, and physical trauma.

MEMORY

Quantum Brain Healing understands the importance of memory in all facets of life. Many illnesses affect memory. There can be memory loss due to partial or complete amnesia. There is often memory loss or poor memory if there is head trauma or brain surgery. This may be due to poor circulation or actual cell death. Memory problems may arise from poor food choices. Vitamin and mineral deficiencies may also be contributing factors.

Extreme trauma or stress or severe anxiety is often a cause of short-term memory problems or problems in the conversion of short-term memory into long-term memory. Side effects of medicine often result in memory problems. Pollutants, toxins, and pesticides can reduce memory. Food allergies can produce memory problems and brain fog. Electromagnetic pollution can impair memory. Poor circulation due to disease or lack of exercise may cause poor memory. There is also an emotional component in memory that differs from person to person.

Anything that increases blood flow to the brain or increases mental activity is capable of increasing intelligence, memory, or concentration.

Quantum Brain Healing uses many ways to increase brain circulation, including herbal formulas, single herbs, acupuncture, music therapy, Hemi-Sync technology developed by the Monroe Institute, nutritional supplements, botanical extracts, food therapy, and nootrophics.

Memory can also be improved with physical activities like deep breathing, yoga, Zen meditation, and exercise. Other activities that stimulate memory improvement include brain exercises, researching on the Internet, card games like bridge and blackjack, and crossword puzzles.

Memory also can be improved by detoxifying heavy metals and chemicals with far infrared sauna, hot yoga, sweat-producing exercise, foot ionizing detox, oral chelation products, and detoxification diets.

Research in sound therapy has focused on the ability of the ear and brain to handle higher frequency than is normal. This can affect learning, memory, and concentration. The therapies that may be included in this area include Metatones, music therapy, sound therapy, Hemi-Sync, Acutonics, Tibetan symbols, and Tibetan singing bowls.

Fluid intelligence is the ability to solve problems or issues by establishing relationships between concepts or ideas where there may have been no previous relationship, knowledge, or skills. It is now possible to increase fluid intelligence, but it is unknown how much memory training or exercise may be required for lasting effects. A number of new software programs are able to achieve this in a cost-effective manner. There are also many types of music and sound therapy that improve fluid intelligence. Listening to many types of music and switching frequently, several times a day on a daily basis, allows new neural pathways to form, and this increases intelligence. Switching any routine on a frequent basis in everyday life will increase the number of neural pathways formed.

Emotional Component of Memory

Emotional blockage can impair brain focus and ability to function. Bach Flower Remedies can be used to reduce and dissipate emotional trauma, stress, and blockages. As the emotions are processed, the brain will perform at a higher level. There is a concept that spending your time with creative, brilliant people will increase your intelligence. It is difficult to prove, because any group of brilliant people would be different, but this is similar to the concept of playing tennis with a better player in order to improve your game. This concept is evident in the music world, in playing chess or bridge, in master painting classes, and in any competitive sport.

Heavy-Metals Poisoning

Heavy-metals poisoning creates many health problems. Toxin exposure may be encountered in bad water, food, air, the workplace, reclaimed soil, toxic waste site, refuse disposal sites, and vaccines. Conditions and diseases related to heavy-metals poisoning may include impaired memory, loss of some cognitive skills, insomnia, depression, anxiety, food allergies. stress, ADHD, obsessive-compulsive disorder (OCD), impaired digestion, neuropathy, colitis, delirium, hallucination, fatigue or chronic fatigue, impaired concentration, brain fog, numbness, hair loss, impaired liver function, lymphoma, auditory problems, cancer, muscle weakness, learning disabilities, dementia, ALS, Parkinson's, certain types of MS, and stupor. Symptoms and diseases vary for different heavy metals.

Research shows that there are heavy metals in the nucleus of many cancer cells. Cancers can go into remission or be cured with detoxification and immune system stimulation. We encounter heavy metals such as aluminum, mercury, lead, arsenic, copper, thallium, and titanium on a constant basis. These metals become more dangerous when heat is applied. An example is aluminum pods for coffee that get heated by hot water as coffee is made. Another example is cans of food or carbonated beverages that get heated in the summer during transport or while sitting in warehouses. This could be a common problem in the Middle East or any desert climate area. Foods that are cooked in older aluminum pots may transfer aluminum into the cooked vegetables. The addition of vinegar to any dish cooked in aluminum may make this worse.

Mercury poisoning can cause social withdrawal or interaction problems, depression, mood disorders, aggressive behavior, OCD, autism, insomnia, delirium, hallucinations, fatigue or chronic fatigue, eating disorders, suicidal threats, ADHD, weakness, colitis, speech problems, difficulty walking, temper tantrums, hearing loss, convulsions, seizures, birth defects, spontaneous abortion, motor problems, rashes, skin problems, nausea, vomiting, diarrhea, stomach cramps, allergies, asthma, and neurological problems.

Aluminum poisoning can cause Alzheimer's, fatigue or chronic fatigue, weakness, dementia, skin problems, rashes, motor disturbances, neurological problems, allergies, asthma, infertility issues, and respiratory diseases.

Lead poisoning can cause memory problems, concentration difficulty, depression, mood swings, irritability, insomnia, sleep disturbance, anxiety, eating disorders, ADHD, mental retardation, impaired intelligence, birth defects, spontaneous abortion, neurological problems, convulsions, seizures, headaches, muscle pain, hypertension, cardiac problems, and suppressed immune function.

The skin is a major organ through which the body detoxifies. Our body also filters toxins from the blood system (detoxification) through the liver, kidneys, gallbladder, and the lymphatic system. It is important to detoxify these systems by drinking plenty of pure water. There are several ways to reduce the heavy-metals load on the body, including diet, nutritional supplements, intravenous chelation therapy, far infrared sauna, foot ionizing detoxification, hot yoga, and any exercise that produces sweat.

There has been a large increase in toxins in many products. The body has a built-in mechanism to help detoxification of heavy metals, but these include eating many raw fruits and vegetables and sweating. People don't sweat as much as they should due to increased use of computers, TV, cars, dishwashers, and other items that reduce physical activity.

Several oral chelation formulas can be purchased at health food stores that reduce heavy metals. The nutritional supplements include cilantro, chlorella, barley, wheatgrass, alfalfa, kelp, alpha lipoic acid, L-cysteine, methionine, vitamin C, garlic, MSM, and pectin.

Glandular Supplements

Porcine or bovine thyroid glandular supplements can be used to improve memory, concentration, and intelligence in people with low or borderline thyroid levels. Porcine glandular supplements are closer to human chemistry than bovine. Thyroid glandular supplements and Armour thyroid can be great to boost healing for chronic sinus or low grade infections that do not resolve after several months of conventional treatment. Thyroid deficiency symptoms include hair loss, constipation, weight gain, susceptibility to infections and illness, brittle nails, depression, memory lapses, concentration problems, irritability, fatigue, low energy, dry or cracked skin, cold intolerance, anxiety, thinning of the outer eyebrows, excessive sleep, low body temperature, low sex drive, and menstrual problems. Successful supplementation should be carefully monitored with frequent basal temperature monitoring or blood tests. Supplements made from animals raised on organic or chemical-free farms are best.

Food

It is important to avoid sugar-laden foods that create significant inflammation in the brain and throughout the body. Chemical additives in water and food should also be avoided. Pure water is a good idea, as dehydration is one of the chief ways that brains become sluggish. Alcohol can destroy brain cells and should be avoided in excess. Alcohol should be avoided, except moderate amounts of low or no-sulfur red wine. Foods that are extremely high in antioxidants are good neuroprotectants.

Food therapy refers to using foods to impact health and body chemistry and metabolism. Food produces a chemical action in the body that can improve aging rates, blood sugar, viral loads, bacteria counts, and digestive speed. This can enhance the brain by increasing clarity, memory, and intelligence. Foods that improve the brain and enhance memory include açai berry extract, blueberries, blackberries, raspberries, cherries, prunes, strawberries, raisins, red grapes, plums, kale, spinach, brussels sprouts, walnuts, almonds, flaxseed, cold-water fish, organic coffee, and organic tea.

Vitamins

Symptoms of vitamin B12 deficiency include fatigue, brain fog, delusion, poor memory, neurological problems, poor concentration, depression, psychosis, irritability, mania, forgetfulness, and increased sleep requirements. These symptoms may also be indicative of other vitamin or mineral deficiencies. Any of these conditions may be treated with B12 if a deficiency exists. Many people have multiple vitamin deficiencies, and all deficiencies must be treated for the patient to heal.

Diseases improved by taking vitamin B12 include long-term memory loss and impaired ability to convert short-term memory into long-term memory. Examine your diet to determine its impact on your B12 deficiency. If you never eat red meat, you are at a higher risk for this deficiency. The brain fog symptom associated with chronic fatigue syndrome can be improved with increased doses of B12. It is always worth noting that digestive problems may be the root of vitamin deficiencies. An HCL digestive enzyme deficiency may also contribute to a B12 deficiency. Consider the use of Life Extension Foundation or Standard Process digestive enzymes. This is especially true for cancer patients and those with auto-immune diseases.

Vitamin B12 is found in beef, caviar, chicken, cheese, eggs, fish, lamb, liver, milk, octopus, and shellfish. A sublingual form of B12 is available. A multivitamin product should also be taken with this supplement so that the other B vitamins do not become deficient. Vitamin B12 is involved in DNA synthesis and fatty acid synthesis, and it helps break down carbohydrates and covert them into energy. It is used by the body to help make several amino acids, including SAM-e. Vitamin B12 is very important for women who are pregnant and suffering from depression or memory problems. Amino acids like SAM-e and GABA are found to change brain chemistry and neurotransmitter levels. The neurotransmitters affected by vitamin B12 directly are involved in learning skills and memory.

Long-term deficiency of omega-3 and omega-6 fatty acids can seriously impair concentration, learning, memory, and neural plasticity. Neurotransmitter and amino acid deficiencies will also result in impaired memory and intelligence. Take high-quality fish oil capsules and eat wild salmon to protect your memory.

Minerals

Boron is a trace mineral found to improve memory. Without the proper minerals, your body will produce insufficient energy to produce optimal health. Boron functions as an activation agent and co-enzyme in your body's metabolism. This most important use of boron in your body is to prevent and reduce inflammation. It also helps the body fight viral infections by increasing the strength of the immune system.

Boron is an antioxidant and is a key anti-aging trace mineral. Boron is involved in Quantum Brain Healing by its impact on hormone regulation. Boron affects key hormones in memory and cognitive thinking. It is involved in mental alertness, manual dexterity, hand-to-eye coordination, attention, perception, short-term memory, and long-term memory. Boron treats memory difficulties and cognitive impairment and helps regulate the levels of calcium, magnesium, and phosphorus. Boron may be found in apples, avocados, grapes, legumes, nuts, pears, plums, prunes, raisins, and tomatoes.

Alpine tea is a drink made from Siberian snow rose and water. Quantum Brain Healing shares this anti-aging drink from the Republic of Georgia, where Alpine tea is sipped on a daily basis with kefir yogurt that contains over ten probiotics. Water in Georgia is glacial water with many glacial minerals. The Siberian snow rose and Alpine tea also are used in Asian hospitals to treat blood pressure problems, dementia, depression, neurosis, psychoses, memory, cognitive difficulties, and concentration problems. The Siberian snow rose has antibiotic properties. It can slightly reduce fat storage, accelerate metabolism, and increase sweating. It is an antioxidant that lowers blood pressure.

It increases blood circulation and passes through the blood-brain barrier. It helps stabilize brain activity and reduces capillary bleeding in the brain - it is unusual to increase brain circulation while reducing the likelihood of capillary bleeding in the brain. The anti-aging protocol of the Republic of Georgia consists of kefir yogurt, Alpine tea, glacial water, local wine, and honey. This anti-aging protocol is very rich in flavonoids.

Most herbal products that increase metabolism are not antioxidants. Snow rose is an exception. Many products what increase metabolism accelerate cellular aging and increase oxidation. It is interesting to note that snow rose has been significantly used in other parts of the world yet it is not well-known. It is not understood if this herb would work this well on people with different genotypes from other areas. People of Russian and Japanese descent should have great success with this product. Many European people have less success with this herb. It is important to use new products under the care and supervision of your health care professional. Quantum Brain Healing shares enthusiasm for the spectacular anti-aging and brain healing properties of Alpine Tea.

Quantum Brain Healing often relies on food-based nutritional supplements for low-toxicity and low-cost healing options. Wild blueberry extract is used in Quantum Orthomolecular Medicine to treat and prevent memory loss. This supplement is a pharmaceutical-grade extract of the active healing ingredient found in food, but it is usually far more concentrated than is found in food. Blueberries are one of the most powerful antioxidants for enhancing memory and preserving brain function. Chasteberry or vitex is a great, inexpensive herb for improving memory. It addresses memory problems due to hormone imbalances.

Nutritional Supplements

Nutritional products that can improve memory are melatonin, lithium orotate mineral salts, CoQ10, phosphatidylserine (PS), DMEA omega-3 fatty acids, choline, piracetam, theophylline, vinpocetine, chlorella, lecithin, galantamine, and spirulina.

Quantum Brain Healing uses several amino acids, separately or together, to improve memory and heal the brain, including acetyl L-carnitine, DL-phenylalanine, GABA, DMAE, L-tyrosine, pregnenolone, and theanine. This concept is amino acid therapy, and the amino acids may or may not be used in large quantities, depending upon the amount of memory loss and how long the patient has experienced memory problems.

Quantum Brain Healing utilizes lithium orotate for treating stress-induced memory loss,

175

kleptomania, schizophrenia, migraine headache, alcoholism, and Alzheimer's disease. Lithium orotate is a trace mineral salt found in RNA and DNA that can travel inside the brain to stabilize many of the chemical activities of the neurons. It protects brain cells in the hippocampus, striatum, and frontal cortex of the brain and helps stimulate the growth of new neurons.

Stress-induced memory loss is often triggered by severe financial loss, job loss, divorce, death of a loved one, living in a war zone, high job stress of a political nature, or bankruptcy of a personal or corporate nature. Lithium orotate can be used to treat neurodegenerative diseases and repair damaged nerves. It is not a pharmaceutical drug that is marketed by pharmaceutical companies. It is one of several trace mineral salts that is commonly used in naturopathic medicine. Lithium orotate can also be used for treating migraine headaches. It is also good for Alzheimer's patients and may help those who have progressed to the point of violent outbursts. It can also be used to treat epilepsy patients. The medical effect in both these diseases is similar and may stem from its ability to stabilize the brain during periods of extremely irregular brain-wave activity.

Lithium orotate also is used to treat alcoholism. Lithium orotate may benefit from its ability to stabilize neurons, grown new neurons, and add to neural plasticity. Lithium orotate might significantly improve the problems associated with alcoholism and allow the patient to progress to the point where other treatments would become an option. DNA and liver function become very damaged by alcoholism. Brain cells may die or decay. Lithium orotate may need to be combined with nutrients that repair and increase the cells' ability to make energy. It may work better in combination with herbs that increase waste removal from the cell.

Lithium orotate can be instrumental in increasing neural plasticity. Increasing your neural plasticity is important for preserving or increasing intelligence. This trace mineral may have a use in treating slow children with memory problems stemming from ADD and OCD.

Herbs

Many health problems are associated with brain issues like memory, brain fog, concentration, and intelligence. In Oriental medicine, these problems are usually connected with blood deficiency, kidney yang, kidney essence deficiency, and qi deficiency. Several Chinese patent herbal formulas work well on memory issues.

The Chinese herbal formulas that treat and heal memory or enhance learning include:

- ➢ Gui Pi Wan improves memory.
- ➢ Ge Jie Da Bu Wan improves memory.

- ➤ Huan Shao Dan Wan improves memory.

- ➤ Ren Shen Shou Wu Pian improves memory.

- ➤ Bu Nao Pian is a general brain tonic that increases brain circulation.

- ➤ Immortal Qi Patent Formula or Bu Zhong Yi Qi Tang He Sheng Mai San Jia Jian by Blue Poppy increases qi and yin to improve memory and intelligence and is anti-aging.

- ➤ Lu Wei Di Huang Tang enhances cognitive ability and increases the speed at which information can be processed. It can increase the speed at which tests can be taken.[1]

- ➤ Turkish Rhubarb Decoction or Rheum Palmatum improves memory, intelligence, concentration, clarity, or focus. This formula has a nootrophic effect: it increases learning and memory ability - it improves the memory acquisition impairments, memory consolidation and memory retrieval induced by scopolamine. It has also been used to treat aphasia, senile dementia, and brain trauma.

Many Ayurvedic and Chinese single herbs improve memory and concentration. These include mucuna pruriens, brahmi, ashwagandha, shankhpushpi (Evolvulus alsinoides), vinpocetine, gotu kola, bacopa monnieri, red panax ginseng, jyotishmati (Celastrus paniculatus), huperzine A, fo-ti, ginseng, ginkgo biloba, Himalayan Rhodiola sacra, he-shou-wu, Jamaican dogwood, sophora, schizandra berry, polygonatum silibicum root, galantamine, sage, rosemary, green tea, mucuna pruriens, yohimbe, bilberry, ginger, kelp, skullcap, shu di huang, rehmannia, betony, peppermint, and morning glory (Evolvulus alsinoides).

Impaired liver function directly affects the brain's ability to think clearly. A common herb called milk thistle is used to detoxify the liver and improve overall liver and brain health. Liver toxicity is a common problem for many people living in metropolitan or polluted areas. Milk thistle is a needed supplement for Quantum Brain Healing. Milk thistle is commonly used for liver detoxification, kidney support, and liver regeneration. The liver is the organ where detoxification occurs on a daily basis.

Wild blueberry extract can cross the blood-brain barrier and target several areas of the brain, including the cerebellum, hippocampus, and cortex areas. The active ingredient in wild blueberry extract is anthocyanin. Wild blueberry extract can improve memory and increase learning ability, as well as increase the brain's ability to make new brain cells. It slows the brain's rate of aging and allows brain cells to stay alive longer. It can reverse aging in the brain - it is an anti-aging supplement that most people can tolerate easily.

Wild blueberry extract causes brains to have higher levels of a brain neurotransmitter called dopamine. Dopamine is the neurotransmitter responsible for controlling body movements and results in better motor control. This extract is an antioxidant and anti-inflammatory. It allows the brain of those with amyloid protein buildup to function more like a normal brain. People with amyloid protein buildups may suffer from dementia and Alzheimer's disease. A great idea would be to include green tea into the diet of this type of patient. Green tea is a cooling substance and calms the brain with theanine, while also increasing brain circulation and fighting virus and bacteria. Its action as a blood thinner can help a brain with amyloid proteins.

Blueberry extract targets oxidative stress and inflammation. Aging of the brain is accelerated by conditions of oxidative stress and inflammation. It is good to include several antioxidants to reverse aging and inflammation. Exercise is extremely important in reversing brain aging. The use of antioxidants shortly after your exercise may enhance their benefits.

Bilberry extract is another product that is an antioxidant and anti-inflammatory. Bilberry can increase the life of your brain's cells. A combination of wild blueberry extract with bilberry extract and green tea can improve an Alzheimer's patient's ability to perform motor tasks. These products improve the brain's ability to convert short-term memory into long-term memory. Bilberry is also a wellness product.

Quantum Brain Healing combines therapeutic doses of amino acids, vitamins, minerals, nutritional supplements, and herbs to treat or heal many brain diseases. Vinpocetine is an herbal extract that is derived from the periwinkle plant. This herb extract has many properties that make it very important in healing the brain. Vinpocetine crosses blood-brain barrier and acts as a neuroprotectant to protect the brain cells and keep them alive longer.

Vinpocetine is an antioxidant that improves brain circulation and metabolism. The extract acts as an anticonvulsant and antismolytic. This anticonvulsant action allows it to reduce seizures in some and prevent seizures in others. This delays the decline for many patients and prevents atherosclerosis when taken on a long-term basis. It slows or prevents abnormal platelet clumping. This is considered an anti-aging brain supplement. Those taking blood thinners should not take vinpocetine. Vinpocetine also should not be taken with large quantities of green tea, due to its blood-thinning properties.

Vinpocetine can be useful for many people in treating ischemia, dementia, Alzheimer's disease, Parkinson's disease, seizures, and memory loss. It can also be used as a memory enhancer for those who need to study seriously, such as older people returning to college. Vinpocetine may be useful in treating epilepsy caused by traumatic injury. This treatment would be best when tried within one to six months after the injury. It would need to be combined with other Quantum Brain Healing therapy.

The European herb piracetam acts upon the brain in many ways, including increasing brain circulation, increasing cholinergic receptors in the brain, enhancing memory, and acting as a neuroprotectant. This actually alters the functioning of the right temporal lobe. Piracetam may be used in treating many brain diseases including amnesia, anxiety, depression, stroke, dyslexia, senility, Alzheimer's, and post-stroke aphasia.

Quantum Brain Healing uses astragalus to enhance immune system resistance and increase physical endurance. This herb improves mental function in one simple way: a stronger body will support a higher-functioning brain. Astragalus is a wonderful, affordable, anti-aging herb that almost everyone can use at some point in their life. Use this herb to fight stress on an occasional basis or to prevent illness. It fights several types of cancer, including small-cell lung cancer, leukemia, and gastrointestinal cancer. It slows tumor growth and prevents the growth of additional tumors. It can increase T-cell activity.

Anyone using this herb for anti-aging purposes should also take food-based multivitamins and change their diet to organic foods, when available. They need to include a yoga or exercise program to help balance neurotransmitters and hormones. A well-planned detoxification program, followed up with bio-identical hormones, is also needed.

Astragalus has antibiotic properties. It is an antiviral, anti-inflammatory, and encourages the body systems to function correctly. It has diuretic properties and increases blood circulation. Many types of blood disease may benefit from this herb. It lowers blood glucose, lowers blood pressure, and enhances cardiac function. Astragalus protects the liver and kidneys. It may be through this action that astragalus helps prevent senility.

Astragalus can be used to treat Alzheimer's disease. It also can improve brain issues connected with chronic fatigue, like brain fog. Astragalus can improve learning and increase memory. It may help patients with diabetes insipidus, a type of brain disease caused by impaired pituitary function. If the pituitary gland is impaired due to inflammation or viral attack, this herb could reverse the condition. Astragalus also can treat dementia and impaired cognitive function.

Although few herbs are able to treat eating disorders, astragalus is the best single herb to handle anorexia. Physical debilitation and brain injury similar to those found in car accidents can be improved for many when astragalus is taken for about two months. Do not take astragalus without informing your health care professional.

Many diseases and conditions are improved by taking hawthorn including memory loss, arteriosclerosis, ischemia, and stroke. Hawthorn is a small berry commonly used to treat heart conditions; it has been used for centuries. Hawthorn also is used for several serious brain diseases. Poor heart function can directly impair the brain by reducing circulation this is a key relationship for anyone with cardiac disease. If there is heart disease, a food-based vitamin and CoQ10 supplement should be added on a daily basis. Hawthorn impacts the brain's circulation, oxygenation levels, and any inflammation.

Hawthorn can cross the blood-brain barrier and affect the brain directly, including increasing blood circulation, lowering blood pressure, decreasing cholesterol, and acting as an antibiotic to decrease bacteria, an anti-inflammatory, or an antioxidant. Hawthorn's ability to reduce cholesterol is connected to its ability to impact arteriosclerosis. A person with brain and heart disease should include mild exercise or a walking plan for an overall strategy to prevent further problems. This person should also take steps to exclude saturated fats from his or her diet and include unsaturated fats. Including salmon in the diet is a great idea.

It is possible that many brain diseases begin when there are heart problems due to damaged heart's failure to properly oxygenate the brain. A heart condition leads to poor circulation, which may increase the amyloid protein buildup in the brain. The other possibility is that impaired circulation increases stress, and the increased stress causes other brain diseases to manifest.

Women and men in their forties and fifties who have memory loss due to hormone imbalances can improve their memory with horny goat weed. This herb balances neurotransmitters and can be used as preventive medicine in families that have multigenerational diseases. The concept involves removing toxins and harmful substances from the body and adding the needed nutritional supplements. The disease is treated by using large amounts of vitamins and amino acids that greatly exceed the normal amounts found in the common diet. Many diseases actually increase the body's requirements for certain vitamins, minerals, and amino acids. The daily recommended levels of vitamins are for a healthy person without a genetic predisposition for a disease. Quantum Orthomolecular Medicine incorporates amino acids with vitamins and nutritional supplements to treat diseases and health issues.

Men and women in midlife experience falling hormone levels and imbalances in neurotransmitters. This is referred to as menopause and andropause (male menopause). The lower hormone levels can create health issues. A combination of amino acids, vitamins, and herbs can often solve or improve these problems. Several herbs can increase hormone levels at this time of life. Some herbs can be taken on a long-term basis, while others should be taken for a shorter time because they produce serious side effects when taken longer. It is important to take the right herbs and monitor the body for any side effects. Monitoring should be done by a health care professional for those with serious illness.

Horny goat weed acts produces testosterone hormone effects in the body that include sexual arousal, libido, increase in sperm count, stimulation of sensory nerves, and increase in desire. It is also used in Asian medicine to treat lower-back disorders like weakness and pain. Its hormone function may reduce inflammation in the lower-back area. It may help older people with their kidney function. It can reduce menopause symptoms in older women. It can increase immune function in elderly patients with a deficient kidney function. It can also strengthen tendons and bones, according to Asian medical use.

In a study comparing horny goat weed to Viagra's drug's active ingredient, a similar function was found in the active ingredient. The drug was slightly stronger at the doses administered, but its side effects can be quite dangerous for those with significantly high blood pressure. Slightly elevated blood pressure may not have the same risk factors. A horny goat weed extract found in the epimedium plant was purified and tested. The extract of horny goat weed increased the levels of a secondary neurotransmitter involved in sexual arousal and libido. Horny goat weed can increase sperm count and sperm motility. It increased nitric oxide, which causes the tissue to relax and directly increases blood flow to the penis and other areas of the body. This action is due to its active ingredient, a flavonoid called Icariin.

If horny goat weed does not improve your hormone levels of testosterone, you may try an amino acid named arginine. Arginine is used to treat erectile dysfunction. Arginine will increase the level of nitric oxide when taken at high levels. The therapeutic dose of Arginine is 5 grams per day. This is a fairly high dose and far exceeds the arginine level found in the normal diet. The reduction of alcohol and recreational drugs is always recommended for those suffering from hormone imbalances or erectile dysfunction. Arginine also functions as a chelator.

Brahmi can help damaged neurons and signaling functions that require time to heal and need biochemical support. It can alter brain speed. The old neural paths become damaged and degraded with aging. Combine brahmi with electro-acupuncture for the best treatment to repair damaged neural pathways. Brahmi is an Ayurvedic herb that improves protein synthesis in brain cell repair and encourages new neuron growth. Implementing acupuncture with herbs and amino acids to stimulate new nerve growth is suggested.

Laser therapy activates the brain's limbic cortex and the frontal lobe. This brain activity resulting from the laser was demonstrated to be faster and more widespread than previously understood. The increased brain activity leads to mood improvement via increased neurotransmitter levels. The limbic and frontal lobes are involved in anxiety, depression, and stress disorders. Laser therapy in the area of the pituitary gland and thyroid areas must be very controlled and should not be overused. The practitioner should not hold the laser directly on top of any endocrine gland.

Several studies have shown that laser acupuncture can benefit memory loss, chronic fatigue, and depression. Laser therapy is the use of a beam of light to stimulate an area of the body or head. Laser results in skin and surface activation occurring along with muscles and tendons. The stimulation of neurotransmitter production is also an important effect. It is unclear how long this treatment's effects last and how many treatments are required for this type of disease.

Memory loss or poor memory is frequently connected to anxiety, depression, and insomnia. Do not ever underestimate the importance of sleep in any illness. Bach Flower Remedies and aromatherapy can help most people gently fall asleep. Try lavender aromatherapy to fall asleep and orange aromatherapy to wake up.

Sex and Memory

Sex improves memory, and this may be due to changes in hormone levels. Research published in 2003 from the University of Calgary (Alberta, Canada) showed that hormones stimulated by sex may cause the production of new brain cells. Sex increases the production of neurotransmitters and hormones, increases the energy level of the brain, increases oxygenation, and increases blood circulation, which are key in the formation of neurons. This may not be true, however, for extremely ill people who have ALS or other diseases resulting in extreme physical disability.

Speed Learning

Another way to improve math, memory, concentration and learning ability from 100% to 600% percent is a program developed called Speed Learning. This would benefit any family with young children or older people re-entering college.

Speed Learning is a technique developed by Professor Lozanov that was distributed in the 1970s by Ostrander and Schroeder. This technology can more than double your ability to learn math, language, and memory skills. The technique has been changed since the early seventies and now includes rhythms and frequencies. The summary of their experiments can be found in the book *Superlearning*. This previously very expensive technology is now available on a CD or DVD at an inexpensive cost of $19.95 plus tax and shipping at the website. The CD or DVD is available in several online locations. This program may be able to raise the IQ by nine points. This programs requires daily sessions for at least one month or longer to impact your brain significantly. The sessions need to be done when your child is not hungry, well hydrated, or tired for the best outcome.

NEUROPATHY

Quantum Brain Healing understands that there are several types of neuropathy. It is essential to get an accurate diagnosis from your doctor prior to exploring alternative medicine therapies for neuropathy. Neuropathy can arise from multiple sclerosis, a brain tumor, diabetes, viral infections, medication side effects, severe hormone or neurotransmitter deficiencies, fatty tumors, cysts, nerve entrapment by bulging disks, physical trauma, and more. Each neuropathy should have the root disease treated.

The neuropathy should be considered a secondary disease or symptom. Diabetics suffer neuropathy caused by elevated blood glucose control levels, which increase oxidative stress and damage nerves. This may be treated successfully with alpha lipoic acid, glutathione, and other antioxidants. Neuropathy caused by a cyst can be improved when the cyst disappears or is surgically removed. Some viruses attack the nerve and impair nerve function, other than MS. These attack specific nerves, like the auditory or optic nerves. Nerves can be impaired by metabolic syndrome. Excess glycation by high blood sugars turns into inflammation. Neuropathy often accompanies autoimmune diseases, such as multiple sclerosis, rheumatoid arthritis, lupus, or Guillain-Barre. This can be improved by aggressively treating the inflammatory condition with nutrition and supplements.

Neurophysiology caused by nerve pressure may benefit from making ergonomic changes in the environment and reduction of repetitive motions or positions. Nutritional deficiency of vitamin B12 and/or folic acid can cause peripheral neuropathy, optic neuropathy, and pernicious anemia. Diabetes causes several vitamin deficiencies that can cause or aggravate neuropathy.

Contact Dr. Heidi Seifert of the Seifert Pain Clinic in Houston for more information on treating neuropathy and pain. Dr. Heidi Seifert is a splendid pain doctor that can treat most cases of neuropathy. She performs surgery at St. Joseph Hospital along with Dr. Bruce Smith. You can also contact Dr. Chuck Brunacardi with Baylor at the Texas Medical Clinic for diabetic stem cell research which may treat diabetic neuropathy.

Quantum Orthomolecular Medicine treats neuropathy that results from heavy-metals toxins and pesticides very carefully. People who have had toxic exposure from lead, mercury, aluminum, titanium, pesticides, plastics, and chemicals must be detoxified in some manner. Far infrared sauna or ionizing foot detoxification can be useful for detoxification purposes. These methods to detox heavy metals usually require from five to ten treatments.

Acupuncture, chiropractic, laser therapy, nutritional therapy, herbs, TENS, herbal formulas, single herbs, yoga, amino acid therapy, magnet therapy, homeopathy, neurobiofeedback therapy, Orthomolecular Medicine, and Alpha-Stim 100 often can help neuropathy.

Acupuncture

Oriental medicine treats peripheral neuropathy as a product of dampness that obstructs the flow of qi and blood in any part of the body. Movement and breath are key to this strategy. The treatment protocol—which includes physical activity, good nutrition, balanced diet, emotional healing, and addressing spiritual issues is to reduce or remove the dampness and increase circulation of the blood and qi. Improving the circulation will improve function and reduce pain. This can be accomplished with herbs and/or acupuncture. There are several different approaches, including scalp acupuncture, auricular acupuncture, moxibustion, electro-acupuncture, cutaneous acupuncture, and body acupuncture. Cutaneous acupuncture involves the use of a special hand-held tool that has small needles attached to a head. This disposable plastic acupuncture device is called a plum blossom needle or seven-star needle. It is used to tap on the skin. Electro-acupuncture uses low frequency stimulation to interrupt the pain signal. The frequency range is usually 2 to 4 hertz.

Scalp acupuncture can be successfully used to treat acute and chronic neuralgia. It is best if used within three months of onset of symptoms. Treatment sessions may last up to one hour. It may take several sessions for an acute problem and two treatments per week for several months to treat a chronic problem. Visit the AOMA and TCTCM student intern clinics in Austin for an affordable treatment plan. Contact Dr. Lisa Lin with TCTCM in Austin at www.TCTCM.edu and Dr. Will Morris of AOMA at www.AOMA.edu. This is the best affordable acupuncture in Texas.

Auricular acupuncture uses several points within the ear, such as neurasthenia, brain, brainstem, spleen, spinal cord, endocrine point, cortex, and subcortex points. This is done with small acupuncture needles or laser acupuncture for between twenty and forty minutes. Neuropathy is a difficult disease to treat, so acupuncture may take up to seven treatments to determine its success.

Moxibustion, or moxa, is a technique that uses the herb called mugwort. The moxa is formed into various shapes—it can be used in a stick form that resembles a cigar or a small solid cone shape placed on the end of the needle. The moxa is lit and heats the needle or the body area over which it is held. This sensation may be localized or can spread superficially or deeper into the body. Indirect moxa is when the moxa is lit and held above a general body area. Direct moxa is when the moxa is placed onto the needle on a specific acupuncture point and then lit. A third type of moxa is liquid moxa, which can be sprayed on to the body and heated with a far infrared heating lamp. This liquid approach is great for people who are allergic to smoke or for large body parts, such as the back. Direct moxa can be used without a needle. Some moxa cones are available with adhesive bottoms. These can be placed on a specific acupuncture point without a needle and then lit.

Acupuncture stimulates the brain to release inhibitory neurotransmitters and opiates that reduce sensitivity to pain and inhibit an overactive nervous system. It also activates nerve receptors that decrease or "gate out" (like a gate being closed) pain signals. Acupuncture increases the production of endorphins in the body, which allows the body to feel better. It reduces inflammation throughout the body. It is able to alter the polarity, change the frequency, and stimulate accelerated removal of cellular debris. This increases the available ATP produced by the mitochondria, allowing more energy, or "qi," to be available for healing purposes.

Food

It is important to avoid sugar-laden foods that create significant inflammation in the brain and throughout the body. Chemical additives in water and food should also be avoided. Pure water is a good idea, as dehydration is one of the chief ways that brains become sluggish. Alcohol is able to destroy brain cells and should be avoided in excess. Foods that are extremely high in antioxidants are good neuroprotectants. Foods that can enhance the brain by increasing clarity, memory, and intelligence include açai berry, blueberries, blackberries, raspberries, cherries, prunes, strawberries, raisins, red grapes, plums, kale, spinach, brussels sprouts, walnuts, almonds, flaxseed, cold-pressed walnut oil, cold-pressed almond oil, seaweed, high-quality whey protein, cold-water fish, Swiss decaffeinated coffee, and organic tea.

Amino Acid Therapy

Quantum Brain Healing uses acetyl-L-carnitine, 5-HTP, GABA, and NAC to help treat and heal neuropathy. These may be needed individually or combined into a protocol. Acetyl-L-carnitine is a neuroprotectant. Recent studies show that acetyl-L-carnitine reduces some chemotherapy-induced and diabetes-induced neuropathy. Amino acid therapy should be incorporated for a minimum of six months. It should be taken in large doses that may be up to six times the suggested amount on the label, two times daily. Depending of the type of neuropathy, this may need to be taken indefinitely. Do not take this large dose if you are also taking 5-HTP on a daily basis.

Acetyl-L-carnitine accelerates nerve regeneration after trauma. This would be useful in neuropathy arising from sports injuries, automobile accidents, household injuries, and wartime injuries. In one study, diabetic animals treated with acetyl-L-carnitine maintained near-normal nerve conduction velocity without any adverse effects on glucose, insulin, or free fatty-acid levels, suggesting that acetyl-L-carnitine can hasten nerve regeneration in the context of diabetes. Acetyl-L-carnitine corrects the altered peripheral nerve function of experimental diabetes. Acetyl-L-carnitine improves nerve conduction velocity and prevents or slows cardiac autonomic neuropathic pain in people with diabetes.

The synthetic pharmaceutical version of GABA has the ability to improve neuropathy in over half of the people with post-herpetic and diabetic neuropathy. The pharmaceutical synthetic version of the main components of GABA are thought to exert their effects of blocking neuropathic pain by binding to the R2-ä subunit of voltage-gated Ca2+ channels. This interaction results in inhibition of calcium influx into neuronal cells. This causes inhibition of neurotransmitter release and suppresses the development of central pain sensitization. It is my belief that the GABA nutritional supplement would support this biochemical action at a lower cost with fewer side effects than the synthetic version. Calcium, magnesium, and neurotransmitter levels imbalances may increase pain due to their connection to calcium ion channels and their affect on the body's electrical circuitry.

Current allopathic treatment for neuropathy includes low-dose tricyclic antidepressants, but these may be ineffective. It is possible to use 5-HTP to change the production and re-uptake rates of neurotransmitters in treating neuropathic pain. This function can also be successfully addressed with the amino acid 5-HTP, which is a precursor to serotonin and dopamine. The 5-HTP should be taken at night and in the morning for a long period. This may mean years of 5-HTP therapy. In some people, 5-HTP supplementation may eliminate the need for medications and can be the sole remedy for neuropathy for some people.

N-acetylcysteine (NAC) is a powerful antioxidant and a precursor to glutathione, an intrinsic antioxidant. NAC can inhibit diabetic neuropathy and protect against chemotherapy-induced neuropathy. This is a powerful amino acid for helping people with chronic fatigue and auto-immune system problems.

Green Tea and Diabetic Neuropathy

Glucose causes excess free radicals and oxidative stress, which leads to inflammation and degradation of nerve fibers. This biochemical action causes diabetic neuropathy and associated pain. Green tea's natural antioxidants can reduce this type of neuropathic damage by blocking free radicals. Green tea also reduces glucose levels and helps prevent or reverse cataracts. It requires five to eight cups of green tea per day to reverse cataracts. Two to three cups per day often will achieve the prevention of cataracts. Green tea capsules are available in regular and caffeine-free varieties, along liquid green tea extracts to put into water or juice. The caffeine free varieties may offer fewer health benefits.

Alpha lipoic acid reduces the onset of diabetes, reduces neuropathy pain associated diabetes, helps control blood sugar levels, and protects the heart, kidneys, and small blood vessels. It also is a chelator of heavy metal toxins. Treatment of symptomatic diabetic peripheral neuropathy with the antioxidant alpha lipoic acid is a long-term proposition. If you have diabetes, you should take alpha lipoic acid. Alpha lipoic acid can delay the onset or the progression of diabetes, and taking it also can reduce the overall cost of diabetes.

Choline is brain food. CDP-choline is a form of choline and cytidine. Choline is a precursor to the phosphatidylcholine (PS). It is used in the structure and function of cells. It is a precursor to acetylcholine. CDP-choline affects neurological functions. Its actions include crossing blood-brain barrier, acting as an antioxidant, and acting as an cognitive enhancer. It enhances immune function and is neuroprotective and cytoprotective. It improves neurological function in an overstressed person and helps balance the brain to improve insomnia.

The cause of diabetic neuropathy is probably the effects of a chronic deficiency of prostacyclin and prostaglandins. The diabetic patient is unable to convert the essential fatty acid (EFA) linoleic acid into gamma-linolenic acid (GLA). This is due to insufficient delta-6-desaturase enzyme. In more severe cases, the EFA metabolism is broken in two places, which is caused by a production deficit of the delta-5-desaturase enzyme farther down the conversion chain. Supplementation of gamma linolenic acid (GLA) is required in order to avoid neuropathy. Increase raw foods in your diet to increase enzyme levels for conversion.

GLA improves diabetic neuropathy. A good source of GLA is evening primrose oil (EPO). It takes about two months for the EPO to have an effect on reducing neuropathy pain. Other forms of GLA include borage oil and black current seed oil. People with mild diabetic neuropathy who receive 480 mg GLA daily have good results. Prostacyclin levels can increase with ginkgo biloba extract, vitamin C, EPA from fish oil, and vanadium.

The omega-3 fatty acids are found in high quantities in cold-water fish such as salmon and are widely consumed for their anti-inflammatory powers. Omega-3s are essential fatty acids and are important components of cell membranes, including the delicate myelin sheath that protects nerves. Studies have shown that omega-3 fatty acids, including eicosapentaenoic acid (EPA) and docosahexaenoic acid (DHA), are able to reduce demyelination in the nerves of diabetic animals, which reduces neuropathic pain.

Alcoholic neuropathy can often benefit from combining benfotiamine, the fat soluble form of vitamin B1, with vitamin B6 and vitamin B12.

Vitamin B6 inhibits a major risk factor for developing diabetic neuropathy. Diabetes patients with neuropathy have been shown to be deficient in vitamin B6 and to benefit from supplementation. Neuropathy caused by vitamin B6 deficiency is indistinguishable from diabetic neuropathy. These vitamin deficiencies may arise from digestion problems, so digestive enzymes should be added.

Sublingual methylcobalamin vitamin B12 or injected vitamin B12 can treat neuropathy caused by B12 deficiency, the symptoms of which include numbness of hands or feet, pins-and-needles sensations, or a burning feeling. B12 can be taken as a preventative for diabetics who have not yet developed this symptom.

Insulin facilitates the transport of vitamin C into cells, decreasing capillary permeability and improving wound healing. Diabetes depletes intracellular vitamin C, which deprives a diabetic of vitamin C's cellular protection. Vitamin C deficiencies exist in many diabetic patients, even as diabetics require a significantly higher level of vitamin C.

Vitamin E can reduce free radicals and oxidative stress. High doses of vitamin E can treat mildly to moderately damaged nerve function from oxidative stress. Use the natural form of this vitamin for best results. Synthetic vitamins are less absorbable and are less bio-available in the cell for metabolism. They are usually more inexpensive.

Coenzyme Q10 or CoQ10 is a ubiquinone. It is a cofactor in the energy production. It is a coenzyme used in energy production by the mitochondria. CoQ10 affects many neurological functions. It is best taken with food that contains some type of lipid or fat. It should be taken in large amounts for neuropathy at the same time as alpha lipoic acid is taken with pure water. It should be taken for several years to see the full effect and obtain all its benefits. It is active in the central cortex of the brain. It enhances immune function and is an antioxidant. It protects brain cells and protects pancreatic beta cells from type 2 diabetes. It crosses the blood-brain barrier. It will help increase energy production by the cell and reduce your fatigue. It helps protect memory loss. It can help neuropathy and other brain diseases like ALS and reduce the frequency of migraine headaches. It delays the onset or delays the progression of Parkinson's, Alzheimer's, ataxia, and ischemia.

Herbs

Curcumin is a neuroprotectant for diseases of the central nervous system. Curcumin has also shown potential in treating diabetic neuropathy and as a neuroprotective agent in central nervous system diseases. This herb is also a spice that can be used in cooking.

Capsaicin is extracted from hot peppers and often placed into a cream or lotion. It can also be

188

taken orally in capsule form. It treats chronic pain by reducing the stimulation of pain receptors. Some people are allergic or sensitive to the cream. Test this cream in a small area of the skin for allergic reaction or sensitivity to see if there is an adverse reaction. Be careful using this cream to reduce diabetic neuropathy pain. The pain crème will be absorbed by your hands and get onto anything else that you touch. Keep the cream away from your eyes.

Physical Activity

Physical activity can improve blood flow to the area of neuropathy and prevent further damage to the area. Good examples of appropriate physical activity include yoga, meditation, karate, aikido, tai chi, qi gong, swimming, walking, rebounding, and ballet. Doing some type of exercise or physical activity every day is essential to reducing neuropathy pain. Any exercise should be mild to avoid nerve injury. When weight lifting, use extreme caution not to overload, which could further worsen the neuropathy pain. Lift light weights.

Yoga

Yoga is a great way to increase circulation, improve flexibility, reduce stress, balance hormone function, restore proper sleep cycles, and improve energy flow. The various types of yoga all offer health benefits.

Power yoga is aerobic in nature and will burn more calories and improve circulation more quickly. It requires that the participant be healthy. A yoga posture, or asana, may be repeated quickly several times. There are standing and floor postures. Power yoga classes usually last one hour.

Hatha yoga increases balance, flexibility, and fitness at a gentle pace suitable for almost everyone. People of ages and levels of fitness can do this yoga. It is very important to discuss all health problems with the yoga instructor prior to class so you can be guided in which postures need to avoid for specific health concerns.

Bikram yoga, or hot yoga, is a great way to detoxify, increase flexibility, and increase metabolism. This practice involves performing yoga postures for ninety minutes in a heated room. The first half of the session involves standing postures, while the second half is floor postures. Because muscles are warm, most people are able to increase flexibility at a faster rate. It is important to take water with you to class. Do not push yourself in this class until you are experienced in how the heat will affect you. Do not do this yoga every day, as it can result in electrolyte imbalances. If you are feeling dizzy after class, replenish your electrolytes with a supplement.

If you have arthritis or other motion-limiting issues, herbs can improve your yoga practice. Herbs can increase flexibility, promote circulation, and stimulate the movement of energy. Herbs can aid in the proper performance of postures by improving circulation, joint function, balance, and coordination. They may be referred to as anti-rheumatic or anti-arthritic agents.

They are mainly herbs for Hatha yoga. The use of herbs in a yoga practice is to reduce limiting factors like sports injuries, neuropathy, arthritis, and other motion limitations. It is not to abuse the body and over-extend muscles or ligaments during practice by those in aggressive practices like competitions. Herbs that can be used in this fashion include adaptogenic herbs such as ashwagandha, panax ginseng, and huang qi. Other herbs used to improve circulation or flexibility in people with arthritis or motor-limiting issues include guggul, shallaki, myrrh, nirgundi, turmeric, saffron, curcumin, sage, salvia, Siberian ginseng, green tea, guarana, Bacopa monnieri, ginkgo biloba, angelica, kava kava, and dasha mula. Avoid over stressing your body through the use of herbal enhancements to push your body beyond its safety zone. There are herbal extracts and essential oils that may be used to help your muscles recover more quickly from power yoga and yoga competitions.

Yoga is an amazing tool for athletic people to manage chronic pain. Professional athletes often have success in using Bikram yoga to replace strong pain medications for solving chronic pain after the muscle or ligament tears have healed. For some people with arthritis or other motion-limiting issues, herbs can improve their yoga practice and take it to the next level. Herbs can increase flexibility, promote circulation, and stimulate the movement of energy. Herbs can aid in the proper performance of postures by improving circulation, joint function, balance, and coordination. Herbs that are adaptogens can help many people in their yoga. Contact an herbalist.

Several yoga poses are wonderful for helping to calm the body. These poses include Downward Facing Dog, Cat Pose, Child Pose, Easy Pose, Head to Knee Pose, Corpse Pose, and Fire Log Pose.

Bio-mat

The Bio-Mat is a device that uses far infrared and amethyst crystals. The patient lies in the mat for twenty or thirty minutes and listens through earphones to sounds and instructions. It seems like a meditation session, and it relaxes your body and the infrared speeds the elimination of toxins. It also ionizes your body with negative ions, which improves your body's ability to heal.

Binaural Beat, Hemi-Sync or Metatone Therapy

Quantum Brain Healing may treat and improve two types of neuropathy. It could help neuropathy due to chronic pain, where the brain circuits are altered, but it will not work for neuropathy caused by tumors or diabetes. The brain biofeedback therapies discussed here will not alter or diminish neuropathy that is caused by a tumor or diabetes. Hemi-sync is a very unusual form of brain biofeedback that synchronizes brain waves and could alter the brain-wave activity and balance between the left and right hemispheres to increase peak performance level. Hemi-Sync reduces mental impairment of almost any type, as well as imbalances in the brain waves that need correction. This can be achieved through extended exposure to the proper frequencies with a binaural beat. Binaural beats occur when different frequencies are delivered to the right and left hemispheres of the brain simultaneously.

Hemi-Sync signals contribute to a greater balance of activity of right and left hemispheres and cortical and subcortical areas of the brain. Hemi-Sync involves binaural beating, a sensory-information stimulus, and changes the information sent to the reticular-thalamic activating system, which improves attention, focus, and level of awareness. Binaural beats are also studied for their influence on the brain, for their ability to entrain brainwaves, and their ability to be used for relaxation and health benefits. Hemi-Sync may enhance IQ for those suffering from extreme stress and anxiety to the point of interfering with their problem solving ability. This is based upon the concept that brain disabilities and impairments are due to emotionally altered vibrations from your mind. These alter the auric energy field of your brain in a negative way to change the type of brain wave or to make the pattern of any type of brain wave irregular.

Magnet Therapy

Magnets relieve pain by relaxing the capillary walls of blood vessels that increase blood flow to the area of pain. They help prevent the muscle spasms that interfere with muscle contractions. They also affect neurotransmitters and neural pathway transmission. Not all people can apply magnets directly to the head because of their hair. Magnets that are imbedded into a hat or headband or other nonadhesive application are required for people with hair. Medical magnets range in shapes, sizes, strengths, and price. For best results, se a coin-shaped neodymium-boron magnet. Neo-magnets are long-lasting and are relatively inexpensive. Medical magnets range in strength from 450 gauss to 10,000 gauss. The higher gauss magnets are more expensive. New York Medical College, Valhalla, researched magnetic foot liners to determine effectiveness in reducing numbness, tingling, and pain associated with diabetic neuropathy. They are often effective in pain relief for neuropathy. Magnets can speed the body's healing capability in many people with muscular or neurological problems.

DMSO

Dimethyl sulfoxide, or DMSO, is an older pharmaceutical drug. Doctors in Russia and Europe commonly use DMSO in treating a wide variety of diseases, but it is uncommon in the United States. DMSO was the first non-steroidal anti-inflammatory discovered since aspirin. DMSO is a transdermal agent and is able to penetrate the skin and to transfer other substances into deeper tissue, even the spinal cord. The use of DMSO is controversial, but clinical research conducted in Russia, Iraq, the Unites States, and the Czech Republic shows that it is anti-inflammatory and reduces pain in nerve fibers. It has been used for decades on animals. It has been used frequently as a topical analgesic. In chronic pain cases, it may take six weeks before pain subsides. The Cleveland Clinic conducted research in 1978 and concluded that DMSO brought significant relief to the majority of patients for inflammatory conditions not caused by infection or tumor, in which symptoms were severe or patients failed to respond to conventional therapy. It has been used in treatment of traumatic head injury. It has not been integrated in a big capacity into western medicine. DMSO has a very strong odor and does not smell good. The side effect may be a headache.

Neurofeedback or EEG Biofeedback

Neurofeedback or EEG biofeedback could be used to treat neuropathy due to a brain malfunction rather than a physical issue, such as a tumor, cyst, or tear in the nerve myelin. Neuropathy due to chronic pain could be a pain circuit malfunction and may be helped with this therapy. This may be considered a very unusual use for EEG biofeedback. It is usually used for treating ADHD and other brain diseases, where patients are given instant feedback on their brain-wave patterns and taught to alter their typical EEG pattern to one that is consistent with a focused, attentive state. EEG data is collected from individuals as they focus on stimuli on a computer screen. Their ability to control the stimuli depends upon their ability to maintain a given EEG level. The skill acquired by mastering neurofeedback is able to improve attention and reduce hyperactive/impulsive behavior.

There are twenty years of published research studies and thousands of case histories that document the effectiveness of biofeedback in the treatment of ADD. There have been no published studies that negate the effectiveness of EEG biofeedback. Medical professionals have written books about the benefits of biofeedback for a variety of disorders. Psychiatrists and neurologists have added EEG biofeedback to their practices.

As with any new therapy or alternative treatment, physicians and health care professionals may discourage patients from pursuing EEG biofeedback. There may be a lack of education or experience in EEG biofeedback or neurofeedback, rather than issues regarding the effectiveness of the therapy. If a health care professional or physician disputes the therapeutic value of biofeedback for the treatment of ADD, request an explanation. EEG biofeedback or neurofeedback is useful in treating ADD, MS, migraines, seizures, depression, closed brain trauma, fibromyalgia, and chronic pain.

New Patent Medicine: Neuronotrophic Growth Factors for Neuropathy

A clinical trial is in progress on recombinant synthetic nerve growth factor (NGF) for the treatment of neuropathy. It is believed that exogenous NGF will stimulate regeneration of nerves. If successful, this may be a new way to treat drug-induced neuropathy pain that can occur from antibiotics or chemotherapy drugs. The trial results are unavailable.

It is my belief that stem cells are our best outcome in the future of neuropathy, especially for that caused by trauma or tumors. There is new research in this area. It will be years before it is widely available and it is likely that Congressional hearings will be required in order for insurance to cover this area of medicine. Contact your Senator and Congressman in writing for their support in funding this area of research. For now, it remains an area of medicine that is available for wealthy individuals and those involved in clinical research trials.

Contact the office of Dr. J. Killian or Dr. Chuck Brunacardi with Baylor in the Texas Medical Center in Houston to discover when this will be offered to patients. Dr. Brunacardi has conducted stem cell research for many years.

OBESSIVE-COMPULSIVE DISEASE

Quantum Brain Healing recognizes that obsessive-compulsive disorder (OCD) is one of the more difficult diseases to treat. Many of the symptoms of this disease are also symptoms of other diseases. OCD sufferers are usually intelligent, highly ethical, and dependable people. They usually are isolated by their condition. Those with OCD learn to hide their symptoms and are afraid of ridicule by those who will not understand their condition.

Symptoms of this disease may include repeatedly doing things like locking doors, washing hands, setting the alarm, cleaning the counter, emptying the trash, setting the correct temperature on the oven, and checking the clock in the middle of the night. Those with OCD may rearrange the kitchen cabinets so the cans of food are in alphabetical order, and they get extremely upset if this is done incorrectly. They can overreact to a speck of dirt on the floor or germs on someone's hand that touches their plate.

This illness may be misdiagnosed as schizophrenia, mania, or bipolar disorder, but OCD is more easily successfully treated than the other diseases when you locate and remove its underlying stressors. These stressors may include bad marriages, alcoholism, rape, or physical abuse without a safe haven, children pornography, child abuse, custody battles of children, poisoning, extremely poor diets, and extreme environmental pollution, such as in Los Angeles or Mexico City. The patient needs to be involved in activities that he enjoys and should focus on a hobby or passion to redirect his energy. OCD can be triggered by unusual circumstances and run-ins with abusers of power and money that target people or companies and invade their privacy and space such as firms working in intelligence or military projects overseas. Men working in a wartime environment may be put into this type of circumstances.

The character of Felix Unger in *The Odd Couple* is an example of someone with OCD tendencies. Billionaire Howard Hughes may have suffered from OCD at some point in his life. Extremely brilliant and inventive, Hughes may have experienced OCD as a result of some airline chemical residue toxin or heavy-metals toxin. OCD can develop from a genetic weakness or a toxic exposure. Years ago, people with OCD might have been called eccentric.

Modern medicine indicates that OCD is largely a chronic disease, but certain examples contradict this idea. Huge amounts of stress can trigger OCD in children, and this would indicate the environmental component of the disease. OCD can start early in life, and early treatment should be everyone's goal. This disease may be triggered by a loss of control; repetitive actions may be the person's attempt to regain control over her environment or body.

The management of dietary sugar intake and eating high-quality protein is very important to managing this disease. Those with OCD would do well with high-quality whey protein, almond milk, almonds, and walnuts for snacks every day. Noted author Dr. Don Colbert suggests combining whey protein with almond milk and drinking it in the morning. Stabilizing glucose metabolism and eating adequate protein will allow patients with OCD to recover more quickly.

In one study, PET scans of patients showed a significant increase in activity in an area of the brain called the right dorsal anterior cingulate cortex, a region involved in reappraisal and suppression of negative emotions. This is the same area of the brain that is affected in anorexia and addiction. Increasing activity in this region corresponded to the OCD patients' improvement in clinical symptoms after a four-week course of intensive therapy. Activity in this area had previously been found to increase after cognitive-behavioral therapy for major depression. Cognitive-behavioral therapy is a great option and is widely available.

The PET scans of OCD patients also showed significant changes in normal glucose metabolism and abnormalities in glutamate, an abundant excitatory neurotransmitter in the brain. This may be normalized with acupuncture and electro-stim acupuncture for some people. The temporal and cerebellum areas of the brain are involved in OCD and where changes have been seen in past studies after longer-term treatment.

OCD sufferers seem to notice a greater improvement with their condition when chemicals in their brain are brought back to normal balance, rather than when behavioral or psychological treatment is used. Liquid amino acids may be helpful for this purpose. Liquid amino acids are not readily available but may be found online. People's Drugstore is found in several locations in Austin, Texas and has a wide variety of liquid amino acids and supplements that are amazing in their range of quality. Visit this store when you are in Austin, Texas. It is my favorite drugstore for alternative medicine products. Another great place to visit if the Herb Bar in Austin for a wide range of essential oils and herbs.

Research indicates that some people are born with a predisposition to OCD. If a family member has OCD, there is a 25 percent or higher chance that other members of the family will develop OCD. The parent who suffers with compulsively pulling out his or her hair may have a child with a 75 percent or higher chance of developing OCD. Those suffering from Tourette's syndrome or vocal tics have a 50 percent chance of having OCD. Tourette's is a physical condition and is not thought to have an environmental component. It does have an emotional component, and most brain diseases get worse when there is stress or trauma.

Serotonin is a neurotransmitter. Neurotransmitters are substances that send signals in the brain. A sufficient amount of serotonin also produces a soothing calming effect to brain activity. The serotonin re-uptake inhibitor function is a way to increase the amount of available serotonin. Antidepressants are serotonin re-uptake inhibitors. Bio-identical hormones, Chinese patent herbal formulas, and amino acids can perform similar actions. Acupuncture, electro-stim, laser auricular acupuncture, and Alpha-Stim 100 can impact serotonin re-uptake in the brain.

Insufficient serotonin is linked with many compulsion issues such as gambling, eating disorders, sugar addiction, alcoholism, anorexia nervosa, self-mutilation, Tourette's syndrome, pulling out hair, and hypochondria. The low levels of serotonin are found in an underactive brain cortex. fMRI images of the brain activity show under-activation in the lateral orbitofrontal cortex and other brain areas. Cognitive-behavioral therapy may affect these areas of the brain after four weeks of daily therapy in patients with obsessive-compulsive disorder. A recently developed neurofeedback software can correct this under-activation in up to 43 percent of the patients.

Drugs or heavy-metals toxins often are the underlying reason for OCD. Quantum Brain Healing begins with detoxifying the body of toxins and heavy metals and follows this with orthomolecular amino acid therapy. Next, it incorporates vitamin IV therapy and acupuncture for twenty treatments. Detoxification may resolve hallucinations for patients with high levels of heavy metals, toxins, and pesticides. OCD may be connected to toxin exposure and symptoms of OCD can improve with detoxification treatments. Hallucinations are not normally part of OCD, rather they may present themselves for OCD patients with serious heavy metal toxins or drug abuse. The patient may get completely well after detoxification and acupuncture. Substance abuse must be eliminated in order for patients to get and remain healthy.

Heavy-Metals Poisoning

Heavy metals poisoning creates many health problems. Toxin exposure may be encountered in bad water, food, air, the workplace, reclaimed soil, toxic waste site, refuse disposal sites, and vaccines. Conditions and diseases related to heavy-metals poisoning include OCD, impaired digestion, neuropathy, colitis, delirium, hallucination, fatigue or chronic fatigue, impaired concentration, brain fog, numbness, hair loss, impaired liver function, cancer, weakness, learning disabilities, dementia, and stupor. Heavy metals cause varying symptoms and diseases.

The nutritional supplements that can remove heavy metals include cilantro, barley, wheatgrass, alfalfa, kelp, alpha lipoic acid, L-cysteine, methionine, vitamin C, garlic, MSM, and pectin.

Heavy metals such as aluminum, mercury, lead, arsenic, copper, thallium, and titanium are encountered on a constant basis. The heavy-metals contamination affects the cells' ability to produce energy, its electrical charge, and its pH level. Some researchers believe that cancer develops from exposure to heavy metals. Normal cells are alkaline, and cancer cells are acidic. Most viruses cannot live in an alkaline state. Cancer cells become dormant at a pH of 7.4, and they die off when the pH reaches 8.5. Some cancers can go into remission or be cured with detoxification and immune system stimulation.

Mercury poisoning can cause OCD, social withdrawal or interaction problems, depression, mood disorders, aggressive behavior, autism, insomnia, delirium, hallucinations, fatigue or chronic fatigue, eating disorders, suicidal threats, ADHD, weakness, speech problems, colitis, difficulty walking, temper tantrums, hearing loss, convulsions, seizures, birth defects, spontaneous abortion, motor problems, rashes, skin problems, nausea, vomiting, diarrhea, stomach cramps, allergies, asthma, and neurological problems.

Aluminum poisoning can cause Alzheimer's, weakness, fatigue or chronic fatigue, dementia, skin problems, rashes, motor disturbances, neurological problems, allergies, asthma, infertility issues, and respiratory diseases.

Lead poisoning can cause memory problems, concentration difficulty, depression, mood swings, irritability, insomnia, sleep disturbance, anxiety, eating disorders, ADHD, mental retardation, impaired intelligence, birth defects, spontaneous abortion, neurological problems, convulsions, seizures, headaches, muscle pain, hypertension, cardiac problems, and suppressed immune function.

The skin is a major organ through which the body detoxifies. Our body also filters toxins from the blood system (detoxification) through the liver, kidneys, gallbladder, and the lymphatic system. It is important to detoxify these systems by drinking plenty of pure water. There are several ways to reduce the heavy-metals load on the body, including diet, nutritional supplements, intravenous chelation therapy, far infrared sauna, foot ionizing detoxification, hot yoga, and any exercise that produces sweat. The skin is a major organ by which the body is able to detoxify.

IV chelation therapy is administered in a doctor's office, usually over several hours. It involves injecting ethylenediaminetetraacetic acid (EDTA) into the bloodstream to remove heavy metals, chemical toxins, mineral deposits, and fatty plaques. EDTA is a synthetic amino acid chelating agent for most metals other than mercury. DMSA and DMPS are chemicals used intravenously to chelate mercury but are not approved by the FDA.

Intravenous Vitamin Cocktail Therapy or Myers Cocktail

The Myers Cocktail is an intravenous therapy consisting of mixing vitamins, minerals, amino acids, and other nutrients. This is very important for everyone suffering from OCD and will increase energy and restore clarity and calmness for many. The B vitamins in it are great for this purpose. One treatment per week for three weeks followed by one treatment per month for three years can improve your health and brain function for those with major disease or toxin exposure. This therapy is widely available in Florida, New York, and California. It is far less available in low income states.

It can be very useful in improving the health of a patient immediately after withdrawal. Most drug addicts are severely deficient in many vitamins and minerals. When nutrients are given intravenously, your digestive system is bypassed and a much higher level of nutrition can be delivered directly to your cells via the bloodstream. The Myers Cocktail improves almost all digestive symptoms, including bloating, diarrhea, food allergies, irritable bowel syndrome, colitis, ulcers, and Crohn's disease.

The Myers Cocktail intravenous therapy improves the body's ability to make energy and increases cellular function. It also increases the rate of excretion of cellular waste to release your toxin load more readily and prevent storage of toxins in your fat. You may feel a warm sensation while the IV is administered. The effect is usually fast, but extremely ill people will require several treatments by physicians or nurse practitioners.

Nutritional Supplements

Choline is brain food. CDP-choline is a form of choline and cytidine. Choline is a precursor to phosphatidylcholine (PS). It is used in the structure and function of cells. It is a precursor to acetylcholine. CDP-choline can affect many neurological functions. Its actions include crossing the blood-brain barrier, acting as an antioxidant, and acting as an cognitive enhancer. It enhances immune function and is neuroprotective and cytoprotective. It improves neurological function in an overstressed person. It helps balance the brain, and this action improves OCD.

Increase your essential fatty-acid intake through fish oil capsules. Take three to four fish oil capsules of a very high quality each day for three to six months—it will take approximately this long before you can determine if any improvement has occurred. If no improvement is seen, eat almonds or walnuts for a morning or afternoon snack for six months. Make sure to monitor your progress or ask someone else to give you feedback.

Quercetin is a bioflavonoid that acts as an antihistamine and can decrease allergic response in the body. It can reduce stress, and anxiety and help prevent prostate cancer. It is an antioxidant and anti-inflammatory. These actions help it reduce inflammation in the brain and improve brain fog.

Alpha lipoic acid increases cellular energy and chelates to remove heavy metals to prevent the buildup of plaque. It improves glucose metabolism. Combine it with CoQ10 and vinpocetine, a blueberry botanical extract, to strengthen the capillaries of the brain and enhance higher thinking. This combination can repair brain problems after taking for two years. Add chorella to further improve nutrition and enhance lymphatic drainage. Lymphatic blockages can cause problems in the body and brain. If you have a lymphatic blockage, decrease dairy consumption and increase your consumption of protein and spring water.

Ketogenic Diet

The ketogenic diet is a high-fat, low-carbohydrate diet with a moderate to high amount of protein. It normally is used to heal and improve epilepsy. This diet also may be helpful for approximately 40 percent of those with OCD. It is not an overnight fix, and it is a difficult diet, but it can moderate electrical activity in the brain if used more than two years. This diet produces an effect similar to starvation and forces the body to burn fat instead of carbohydrates. Calories are strictly controlled so that weight is not lost or gained during the diet. Regular growth and repair of the body continues. The ketogenic diet is heavily supplemented with vitamins and minerals. It should be done under the care of a registered dietician or physician. Fluids are restricted so that electrolytes do not get out of balance.

The ketogenic diet alters the genes involved in energy metabolism of the brain. This action helps to stabilize neurons when seizure activity occurs. The diet increases the energy production in the hippocampus, helps the brain to become more resistant to reduced glucose levels, and increases the brain's ability to handle metabolism changes. When glucose is not sufficient, the body burns fat. The fat is not completely burned, and ketones are formed. The high level of ketones formed seems to reduce or eliminate seizures in many people. People who are unable to control seizure activity can use this diet by other means. People can discontinue this diet after they have been seizure-free for a period of approximately two years.

The ketogenic diet seems to alter the seizure threshold with the elevation of ketone levels. Approximately 40 percent of OCD patients have brains with abnormal brain activity that is similar to those found in seizures. This diet has the potential to treat OCD, Alzheimer's, and Parkinson's diseases. Side effects of the ketogenic diet include dehydration, kidney stones, constipation, vomiting, increased cholesterol, lower growth rate, behavior changes, and mood changes.

NAET

NAET can be used to treat and improve many brain illnesses. Most diseases are impacted by environmental or food allergies. OCD patients should be diagnosed and treated for allergens. This will help their immune system improve and will improve the patient's prognosis. It will not work on all the people. NAET will require about two treatments per week over a period of approximately one year, and the treatments last approximately thirty-five to forty-five minutes. The severity of the case and the age of the patient will determine the number of sessions required.

Nambudripad's Allergy Elimination Technique (NAET) is a technique to eliminate allergies of all types and levels using a blend of medical therapies taken from acupuncture or acupressure, allopathy, chiropractic, nutrition, and kinesiology. It can be noninvasive when acupressure is utilized. It is pain-free, but there may be the presentation of allergic symptoms during the twenty-five hour period following the treatment. The patient needs to be rested and hydrated and not hungry in order for an optimal treatment. There is usually an avoidance period of twenty-five hours after the treatment, where specific items need to be avoided. These items or foods will be identified for the patient at the time of treatment.

One allergen is treated at a time. If you are not severely immune deficient, you may need just one treatment to desensitize one allergen. OCD patients have immune systems that may have been exposed to heavy metals, toxins, recreational drugs, and extreme trauma. Any additional symptoms, such as depression, anxiety, insomnia, memory loss, eating disorders, and alcoholism, will require additional attention and treatment. A person with mild to moderate allergies may take about fifteen to twenty office visits to desensitize fifteen to twenty food and environmental allergens. Basic essential nutrients are treated and cleared during the first few visits. It is important to diagnose and treat the primary allergens that negatively affect the body's ability to maintain health. The longer an allergy goes untreated, the more inflammation occurs. Ordinary items that are not allergens will cause a reaction in a body that is in a state of high inflammation. Extremely ill people with many allergies may require an extended period to get well, but there should be some improvement shown after the initial fifteen to twenty treatments.

NAET can treat many diseases, including brain illnesses, cancer, autoimmune diseases, and diabetes. Diseases improve when NAET is used to reduce allergenic inflammation throughout the body. Chronic illness usually requires more treatments to produce desired results. Acute situations, such as food poisoning, can respond within two hours. The website to locate a trained NAET practitioner anywhere in the world is www.naet.com.

Hypnotherapy

The Mayo Clinic states that hypnotherapy may treat many disease symptoms associated with the brain. It can be used alone or in combination with other alternative medicine treatments. Hypnotherapy can treat some of the odd symptoms and habits associated with OCD. Eliminating even small negative behaviors connected with OCD will improve your prognosis. Hypnotherapy can:

> address binge eating, anorexia, and overeating

> reduce or eliminate fears, stress, and anxiety

> lower blood pressure (dizziness)

> address repetitive behaviors

> reduce the intensity or frequency of headaches, including migraines

> improve smoking and bed-wetting

Hypnosis will help many symptoms but not all, and it does not work on everyone. It requires patient motivation and a well-trained therapist. Hypnosis is a heightened state of concentration that creates deep relaxation and quiets the mind. A hypnosis session usually requires approximately one hour, and several sessions are needed for benefits to be seen.

Insomnia and OCD

If there is a melatonin deficiency, the body's circadian rhythm is imbalanced, and the body will wake up at irregular times due to brain-wave irregularities and hormone imbalances. Melatonin supplements of 1.5 to 3 mg per day, taken for about four weeks, may help this deficiency. A combination capsule containing vitamin D, magnesium, and calcium is another aid for sleep. St. John's wort, hops, valerian, passionflower, chamomile, and lemon balm are herbs that may induce sleep. Bach Flower Remedies are a wonderful, mild tool for helping people relax and can treat insomnia. OCD becomes very problematic when patients get too little sleep. Eight to nine hours of sleep each night is essential for those with OCD. Aromatic essential oils are also a great tool for aiding with sleep. There are small pillows filled with lavender that can be warmed in the microwave to release the aroma. Orthomolecular Medicine can also be used to treat insomnia. The amino acids used may include 5-HTP, theanine, and orthinine.

Try to develop a safe haven to sleep in, where no TV or other activities are allowed. Do not work or eat in your bedroom. Your sleep environment should include cotton, silk, or wool products on the bed.

Amino Acid Therapy

GABA is an amino acid used in the field of holistic healing to treat depression, insomnia, and anxiety. It may be very effective for those people who cannot use antidepressants due to side effects. GABA is an amino acid that is a calming neurotransmitter. It is usually deficient in those with depression and anxiety. GABA may also be useful in treating OCD and insomnia. There are frequently several neurotransmitters imbalances in most brain diseases.

Quantum Brain Healing can treat several addictions with Orthomolecular Medicine. Orthomolecular Medicine for Quantum Brain Healing focuses on using amino acid therapy and antioxidants supplements to heal the brain. Amino acid therapy can help addicts recover from valium, pot, alcohol, and food additions.

Using GABA for addiction issues should be a long-term strategy. This supplement should be added for two to five years. Treating addiction issues with amino acid therapy requires a long-term commitment. Valium addiction frequently occurs due to severe anxiety, and the patient is attempting to self-treat his anxiety or depression. It can help you feel better relatively quickly and should not be thought of as a slow nutritional therapy for mood disorders and brain symptoms. GABA is not effective in treating severe depression or bipolar disorder.

Another amino acid that is used in Orthomolecular Medicine is 5-HTP. This supplement can be used in moderate cases of OCD to calm overstimulated or overexcited nerves. This amino amino acid can be evaluated to replace tricyclic antidepressants for those with OCD. This needs to used on a long term basis. This can be used along with CoQ10 and valerian. OCD patients should seek liquid amino acids and amino acid IV therapy because their digestion may be impaired. They are very good candidates for probiotics and digestive enzymes. The use of either probiotics or digestive enzymes will increase the effectiveness of the amino acid therapy.

Lithium Orotate

Quantum Brain Healing utilizes lithium orotate for treating OCD, ADHD, schizophrenia, migraine headache, alcoholism, stress-induced memory loss, and Alzheimer's disease. Lithium orotate is a trace mineral salt found in RNA and DNA. Lithium orotate increases neural plasticity for preserving or increasing intelligence and helps grow new brain cells. It can be used to treat neurodegenerative diseases and repair damaged nerves. Lithium orotate is not a pharmaceutical drug; it is one of several trace mineral salts that is commonly used in naturopathic medicine. It is not widely available. You may need to look for this online and keep your doctor informed. Print out the product information when you order and mail a copy to your doctor for your patient file. Do not take large amounts of the product. It can be useful for some people in small amounts. Never embark on this therapy without informing your doctor and ask them to closely follow your progress.

Auricular Therapy

Auricular therapy, or acupuncture of the ear, is a way to treat the entire body with acupuncture points located on the ear. This alternative medicine therapy mobilizes endorphins and enkaphlins opioid peptides, increases serotonin and dopamine neurotransmitters, and increases levels of substance P and cholecystokinin (CCK). Auricular acupuncture helps the body to balance levels of stress and sex hormones. It helps reduce cortisol and glucose levels and allows the body to reduce its overall inflammation level. Auricular therapy modulates neurotransmitters and is very helpful in dealing with substance abuse recovery and mood disorders. Auricular therapy can be used in addition to acupuncture on the body and scalp.

Auricular therapy can include needles, electrical stimulation, laser therapy, or electro-acupuncture. Opiate withdrawal symptoms can be reduced within fifteen minutes of application of auricular therapy to certain auricular acupuncture points by applying electrical stimulation to the ear. It can be used to treat cocaine, crystal meth, methadone, morphine, alcohol, opiate, food, sex, and nicotine addiction.

National Acupuncture Detoxification Association (NADA) established five auricular points for treating addiction issues. NADA protocols are offered in over five hundred clinics worldwide, including the United States, Europe, Australia and the Caribbean. Yale University has conducted research on the effectiveness of the NADA protocol for cocaine, heroin, and methadone addiction.

The auricular acupuncture points for treating OCD include:

- Shen Men—stress, anxiety, and excessive sensitivity
- Autonomic Point—balance nervous systems and blood circulation
- Liver—hepatitis and cirrhosis
- Kidney—kidney disorders and heavy-metals toxins excretion
- Cortex
- Large Intestine
- Subcortex
- Zero Point
- Brain

This treatment protocol creates reduced anxiety, improved sleep, fewer cravings, less stress and anxiety, and reduced repetitive behaviors. Patients who successfully completed conventional treatment with the combined with auricular therapy showed the fastest recovery with the highest alcohol and drug abstinence rates.

The highest success rates were those patients who received auricular therapy for five days per week for the first month and three times per week for the second month of treatment. It is relatively low cost and produces very few side effects.

Ozonated Water

Ozonated water could be quite useful for OCD patients. It is obtained via an elaborate water purification system that may be hardwired under the kitchen sink or used next to the kitchen faucet. It produces pure water that has been ozonated and is alkalizing in nature. The water may improve conditions in the body associated with high acidity levels. There is little research on this technology, however, other than that many diseases get far worse with high levels of acidity in the body, including cancer and Alzheimer's disease. Ozonated water may help those with serious viruses and you cannot imagine how this can enhance the body. This type of water may enhance water metabolism through the body and alter energy production rates. This kitchen model machine may cost $1,200 to $2,500.

Herbs

Lemon balm is an antiviral, sedative, and antibiotic agent used to treat moderate OCD, stress, anxiety, or nervous exhaustion. It also lowers stress and anxiety associated with drug and smoking addiction. Lemon balm can reduce brain fog for enhanced learning. Lemon balm can act as an antidepressant for mild depression. Quantum Brain Healing also uses lemon balm to treat primary brain disease or secondary brain symptoms from diseases targeting other body organs.

Lobelia increases norepinephrine release from the hippocampus and stimulates the release of dopamine. It is a sedative, anxiolytic, and enhances cognitive performance. It may be useful in treating OCD, drug withdrawal symptoms, smoking cessation, depression, and headaches. It may also be useful in treating overall inflammation and may delay aging.

Brahmi is an Ayurvedic herb that improves protein synthesis in brain-cell repair and encourages new neuron growth. Brahmi can help treat OCD because it is an adaptogen and supports balance in the cortex.

Metatones Therapy

This is auditory vibrational energy therapy to address problems for those suffering from OCD, ADD, ADHD, insomnia, and PTSD. This therapy allows those with serious brain-wave problems and imbalances between the left and right hemispheres to become balanced after about four months of use. It involves adjusting cellular resonance in the body and brain. This is available online for purchase. There is a new physical fitness equipment device that produce a similar outcome with vibrating plates at variable high speeds, and costs about $9,000 to $30,000 depending upon the level of sophistication of the equipment design. This fitness product can move lymphatic fluid along with increasing blood circulation for amazing results.

Interactive Metronome Therapy

Interactive metronome (IM) therapy was created to improve learning and developmental disorders in children. It is also effective for adults in brain rehabilitation. IM is a neuromotor assessment and treatment tool used in therapy to improve motor planning and sequencing using neurosensory and neuromotor exercises to increase brain plasticity. OCD is a processing disorder and has symptoms that are similar to many of the diseases that have been successfully treated with IM. OCD has genetic and environmental roots, and IM therapy addresses the specific brain areas that are sub-functioning for OCD.

The human brain's efficiency and performance depend on the seamless transition of neuronal network signals from one area of the brain to another. The research of Neal Alpiner, MD, believes that IM works by augmenting internal processing speed within the neuroaxis. The brain is affected in the cerebellum, prefrontal cortex, cingulate gyrus, and basal ganglia. This area is responsible for sustained attention, language formulation, motor coordination, and balance.

The IM program provides a structured, goal-oriented process that challenges the patient to synchronize a range of hand and foot exercises to a precise computer-generated reference tone heard through headphones. IM requires a series of twelve to fifteen sessions. It works through listening to a rhythmic sound through stereo headphones and responding by tapping or clapping and attempting to match the beat. A patented auditory-visual guidance system provides immediate feedback measured in milliseconds, and a score is provided.

IM trains the brain to learn rhythm and timing. As timing improves, so do motor control, coordination, focus, concentration, language processing, aggression, impulsiveness, endurance, strength, filtering out distractions, attention span, self-control, school performance, and social performance. IM has been used to treat dyslexia, sensory integration disorder, ADHD, traumatic brain injury (TBI), cerebral vascular accident (CVA), nonverbal learning disorder, Asperger's syndrome, delayed speech development, Parkinson's disease, and balance problems.

Reclaimis Medical Device for OCD

Reclaimis is a new device by Medtronic with FDA approval. It is the first implantable deep-brain stimulator for severe obsessive-compulsive disorder. It is implanted in the torso near the abdomen, and four electrodes are wired to the brain. Electricity pulses block abnormal nerve signals in the brain and improve or heal OCD symptoms that drugs or psychotherapy failed to treat. It is a treatment, however, and not a cure at the present time. When the abnormal brain signals are normalized for a long period of time, the brain may be able to heal itself. The brain neurotransmitters will change and make normal neurotransmitter levels. Moods and anxiety are better after use, but this may take years to accomplish. It may be accomplished more quickly if other therapies are added. The Reclaimis medical device should not be used for those requiring electro-convulsive shock therapy (ECT) or anyone having magnetic resonance imaging or diathermy.

Alpha-Stim 100

This small medical device is prescribed by doctors and acupuncturists; it is slightly larger than a deck of cards. It has wires that attach to ear clips. Each ear clip has a small pad where several drops of a liquid are placed before the clips are attached to your earlobes. The time and frequency are set at your prescribed levels. The device operates with a D battery and may be worn several times per week. This should be tried for no more than seven to nineteen minutes during its initial use. If there is pain, lower the frequency setting. If this does not remove the pain, discontinue wearing the device and inform the doctor immediately. It has not been tested for this use. The Alpha-Stim 100 is able to affect the brain in many ways and is being used in some VA Hospitals for several brain conditions. It is very good at altering neurotransmitter levels and has been tried on seizures. The device can replace antidepressants for those suffering from depression. If you have a brain disorder like Alzheimer's or epilepsy and have the co-morbidity of depression, drug interactions for two or more diseases can cause side effects that cannot be predicted. This device can help eliminate one of your medications and reduce drug interactions and drug side effects to improve your health.

NEUROCARE NC10004PXP

This amazing medical device, a therapeutic electric stimulator, is based on patented technology and should never be confused with neurofeedback devices or brain stimulating devices. The system has a low-amperage technology. It can be used to treat many brain illnesses, including OCD, Alzheimer's, deep depression, insomnia, anxiety, shopping addiction, drug addiction, gambling addiction, and other addictions. Its other medical uses include diabetic wound care, muscle atrophy, paralysis from trauma, post-surgical recovery, prevention of deep vein thrombosis, and increasing local circulation. The treatment of OCD requires four to twelve sessions. After the initial treatments with this device, evaluate your treatment results. If you have more than one brain disease, get evaluated after only four treatment sessions with the device. Make sure that a licensed psychiatrist or neurologist performs your evaluation if you have several brain disease. You can get worse when over-treated. An example of this case is a Parkinson's patient suffering from OCD and depression.

Look carefully for any unexpected personality changes or other health changed during this period. Do not overuse this device. This is not like the Alpha-Stim 100 and should not be considered a long term device to replace medication or be used to treat more than one brain disease or illness without a pet scan or fMRI or other high level expensive diagnostic brain test. It can be dangerous if used too often and the changes are permanent.

Additional sessions may be needed, depending on the length of time the person has had the disease, for a minimum of twelve months' treatment. It is possible to notice improvement after a single session. The equipment is not inexpensive. It is fairly user friendly and the device may be leased from doctors for home use if long-term use is required.

Oxytocin Hormone Therapy

Oxytocin hormone therapy is very new. Oxytocin is a hormone and neurotransmitter produced by the anterior lobe of the pituitary. This therapy can be dangerous if used incorrectly. This hormone affects your ability to maintain healthy interpersonal relationships and personal boundaries. Oxytocin can be utilized in OCD to reduce repetitive behaviors. Research at Emory University shows that the hormone administered intravenously has a positive effect in reducing repetitive behaviors and anxiety. It must be used carefully, as it has negative effects on memory and learning. Use this hormone for a short time and monitor very closely.

Intranasal oxytocin administration reduces stimulation of brain circuits involved in fear, increase levels of eye contact, and increases both trust and generosity. This hormone may indirectly increase carbohydrate metabolism. Patients receiving oxytocin hormone do not notice feeling different, but they have altered responses and reactions. Oxytocin reduces cocaine, morphine, heroin, and sweets cravings and reduces symptoms of drug withdrawal. Oxytocin inhibits the development of tolerance to opiates, cocaine, alcohol, and reduce withdrawal symptoms in animal studies. Pursue this with caution. Most of the research has been on animals. Do not travel overseas for more aggressive treatment with this therapy. Find an experienced research health care professional with this specific area of expertise and associated with a major medical institution. Contact USC, Vanderbilt, or Emory University to speak with their researchers.

Homeopathy

Homeopathy seeks to stimulate the body's defense mechanisms and processes so as to prevent or treat illness. Homeopathy uses a diluted substance to treat a person. This dilution, or "remedy," would cause the illness or symptom if given at full strength. There is debate among alternative medical practitioners on why homeopathy is successful for some people, while it has little or no effect for other. The varying outcomes may be affected by the strength of the person's immune system.

There are a number of different homeopathic remedies that treat a disease and are differentiated by symptoms. Focus on finding a knowledgeable practitioner. Discontinue taking the remedy if there has not been improvement after one month and/or seek another opinion.

A visit with a medical practitioner that has some training in homeopathy would prevent mistakes. Many homeopathic remedies treat overlapping symptoms. If you reside in an area without a homeopathic doctor or naturopathic doctor who uses homeopathy, contact King Homeopathy in Asheville, North Carolina, for help obtaining the remedies and a specialist. Additional options for obtaining homeopathic products include online stores and various natural food stores, such as Whole Foods or Central Market. Some homeopathic practitioners custom-make remedies for each person. Some computer medical devices can produce homeopathic remedies. The list below sets out remedies and the symptoms that they treat:

- Agaricus muscarius — epilepsy, multiple sclerosis, chorea, senile dementia and tremors associated with alcoholism
- Aluminum oxydatum — dizziness, multiple sclerosis
- Aranea diadema — neuralgia, insomnia in alcoholics
- Avena sativa — mental exhaustion
- Bufo — epilepsy
- Coffea cruda — excessive mental activity, insomnia
- Crocus sativus — possible schizophrenia
- Delphinium staphisagria — neuralgia
- Hydrastis canadensis — epilepsy
- Hyoscyamus niger — epilepsy
- Kalium bromatum — nervous system disorders, epilepsy
- Moschus moschiferus — dizziness, neurosis
- Mygale lasiodora — anxiety, restlessness
- Nux moschata — mental illness, hysteria, epilepsy
- Picrinicum acidum — severe mental fatigue, possibly due to grief
- Plumbum metallicum — multiple sclerosis, Parkinson's
- Spigelia anthelmia — migraine, neuralgia
- Stannum metallicum — neuralgia, nervous disorder

➤ Tarentula cubensis	deliriousness, restlessness, physical pain during extended death	
➤ Zincum metallicum	extreme mental exhaustion, brain fatigue, irritability, jumpiness	

POST-TRAUMATIC STRESS DISORDER

Quantum Brain Healing can be used for traumatic brain injury patients having terrible memories that continue for decades. Quantum Brain Healing is the use of alternative medicine and Orthomolecular Medicine for a directed change in brain chemistry. Traumatic brain injury may occur in a sports injury, such as professional football or baseball. It may also be a common problem associated with serious automobile accidents or falling from a roof when removing Christmas lights. This trauma can also occur for victims of violent crimes at home or the office.

The brain is constantly changing, and when it forms a memory, suffers from stress, or catches a disease, the brain metabolism and neurotransmitters change. These brain changes alter the signals and information transmitted to the brain. This is referred to as neural plasticity. When false signals are transmitted or information flow is impaired, neural plasticity is reduced. Neural plasticity is reduced in post-traumatic stress disorder (PTSD). One of the keys to treating PTSD is expanding or increasing neural plasticity.

PTSD and traumatic brain injury patients experience memory impairment, including not remembering aspects of the trauma or entire events. Their trauma is stored on a cellular level, and their memory loss does not reduce emotional trauma or physical symptoms.

Their brain dysfunction impairs the amygdala and hippocampus areas until it has been repaired. The hippocampus is essential to connecting and organizing different aspects of a memory and is largely responsible for tracing the memory of an event to its time, place, and circumstance. Damage to the hippocampus often results in incomplete or delayed recall of an abusive or traumatic experience. If the damage to the hippocampus is repaired, the memory may be partially restored, but this may never occur.

Several neurotransmitters are involved in PTSD or traumatic brain injury, including serotonin, noradrenaline, and dopamine. The hypothalamic-pituitary-adrenal (HPA) axis suffers damage after serious brain injury or PTSD. The neurotransmitter receptors are overactive. This can cause higher levels of noradrenaline and increased autonomic activity.

Dopamine and noradrenaline are the neurotransmitters associated with motivation. Dopamine imbalances may cause situations where there is an inability to derive pleasure from a normally happy situation. Complex thinking, emotions, and moods are affected by dopamine, serotonin, and noradrenaline. Noradrenaline and serotonin affect anxiety and irritability levels. Serotonin is connected to fear conditioning, stress-induced corticosteroid release, depression, anxiety, impulsiveness, body temperature, pain feelings, sleep regulation, mood relation, hormonal activity, and aggression. Small problems result in increased noradrenaline levels.

Alternative therapies for PTSD include acupuncture, electro-acupuncture therapy, scalp acupuncture, ear acupuncture, laser acupuncture, NAET, Chinese herbal formulas, single herbs, botanical extracts, Bach Flower Remedies, music therapy, yoga, tai chi, medical qi gong, BEST, EFT, massage therapy, reflexology, cranial sacral therapy, animal therapy, far infrared sauna, detoxification, vitamin IV therapy, orthomolecular amino acid therapy, food therapy, dietary changes, addiction treatment, hyperbaric oxygen therapy, guided imagery, Hemi-Sync, vibrational medicine with pulsed energy machines, hypnotherapy, and ionizing foot detoxification.

Sexual dysfunction is often found in those suffering from traumatic brain injury and PTSD. Horny goat weed and deer antler herbal products may be useful to balance hormone levels and endocrine levels for sexual dysfunction in men. This will take from four to twelve weeks. Both herbs increase testosterone and alter serotonin levels. Amino acids can also quickly alter neurotransmitter levels to help stabilize this disorder.

Traumatic brain injury and PTSD patients experiencing stress may have increased response to dopamine agonists like cocaine. PTSD patients experiences hyper-vigilance or paranoia that may be mediated by the dopamine system. The PTSD body produces opioids during trauma that function like internal painkillers. PTSD patients have an overactive nervous system that requires less intense shock to cause trauma. Opioid substance abuse is often reported by patients with PTSD. The opioid blocker naloxone may reverse the analgesia induced by stress.

Cortisol levels seem unstable in these patients, and low cortisol levels may occur. This can be caused by hyper-suppression of cortisol. PTSD and traumatic brain injury may cause increased secretion of corticotropin-releasing factor (CRF). This type of stress on the body seriously alters hormone and neurotransmitter levels. After the brain is balanced for a significant period, the frequency of traumatic memories and physical symptoms will diminish. Quantum Brain Healing for this type of patient will often require amino acids, herbs, vitamins, and antioxidants. These products may be combined into an IV for faster results. This IV drip will take approximately one to two hours in a doctor's office. The patient may feel the difference within hours. A minimum of five to twelve sessions of the IV drips should be used for a severely ill person.

There may be overlap in diagnosis and treatment of veterans and abused children. Brigham Young University researchers found a reduction in size of the hippocampus occurs after stress or trauma in childhood. This supports the argument that shrinkage of the brain's hippocampus is similar to PTSD or stress exposure. PTSD patients have traumatic memories that continue for many decades, are easily triggered, and seem overwhelming in nature. PTSD patients experience memory impairment, including not remembering aspects of the trauma or entire events. Their trauma is stored on a cellular level, and their memory does not reduce emotional trauma or physical symptoms. Their brain dysfunction remains in the amygdala and hippocampus areas until it has been repaired.

Child abuse is the most common cause of PTSD, but many other psychological traumas can cause the disorder, such as car accidents, adoption, military combat, rape, and assault. PTSD can include repetitive memories of the event, nightmares, flashbacks, increased aggression, relationship impairment, problems with memory and concentration, fragmentation of memory, dissociation, anxiety, and small events triggering immediate panic or substance abuse. Abused children need to be diagnosed and treated for PTSD. They also need to be examined for depression and treated immediately.

The hippocampus is involved with emotion, mood, learning, and memory. PTSD may cause atrophy of the hippocampus and negatively affect memory, learning, and moods. Veterans returning to campus after service may need to pay special attention to this issue. It can be solved and reversed with the therapies and techniques listed in this chapter. Yale University research suggests that the stress of PTSD may extend to the entire endocrine system. Uncontrolled stress may result in shrinkage or damage of the entire brain and many of the endocrine glands. This would be caused by increased inflammation, increased blood pressure, and diminished circulation.

Stress decreases the production of vascular endothelial growth factor (VEGF) by the hippocampus. Stress impacts emotion, mood, learning, memory, and causes the atrophy and loss of brain cells in the hippocampus. Stress can cause depression, which also results in decreased production of VEGF. Antidepressants can produce increased production of VEGF and an increase of neurons. Amino acids and nootropics can produce a similar outcome of increasing neurons and increasing cognitive ability. Maintaining optimal levels of excitatory amino acid and serotonin prevents neuron death and cognitive impairment.

Several neurotransmitters are involved in PTSD, including serotonin, noradrenaline, and dopamine. The hypothalamic-pituitary-adrenal (HPA) axis suffers damage in PTSD. The neurotransmitter receptors are overactive. There may be higher levels of noradrenaline and increased autonomic activity. Serotonin is involved in stress-induced corticosteroid release. Small problems like getting stuck in traffic for an hour or losing your vacation day at work can result in increased noradrenaline levels. Your entire endocrine system can suffer and more than one of your hormones can become unbalanced due to this type of stress.

PTSD patients experiencing stress may have increased response to cocaine. Those with severe stress and trauma seek drugs and alcohol more often than their healthy counterparts. Their cocaine response is due to reduced levels of dopamine caused by the PTSD or brain trauma. They may have symptoms of depression, moodiness, pain, or paranoia due to their dopamine shortage that gets dulled by the cocaine or opiate. This occurs through the body's production of opioids during trauma in order to act as internal painkillers. PTSD allows their bodies to over react and this patient then requires less intense shock for subsequent analgesia. Opioid substance abuse is often preferred by patients with PTSD over other types of drugs. The opioid blocker naloxone has been reported to reverse the analgesia induced by stress.

PTSD patients have unstable or low cortisol levels and increased the secretion of corticotropin-releasing factor (CRF). This causes increased negative feedback and decreases the body's ability to adapt to stress. The hormone system in PTSD can be conceived as overly responsive or sensitized.

Fear is a key issue for child abuse, trauma, physical abuse, emotional abuse, sexual abuse, and war. This type of event triggers a fear response and heightens the fear response for other smaller issues that can arise. PTSD patients experience less pain sensitivity, a pattern that may be related to altered pain processing in the brain. They also show altered processing of moods. Research indicates that the amygdala plays a key role in fear and anxiety and is overactive in PTSD. PTSD patients experience extreme emotional swings and lowered physical sensation.

Patients with PTSD most likely have altered amygdala processing function. PTSD patients have higher than average heroin addiction rates. People who experience high levels of fear and violence in war become addicted to the heightened emotions that heroin allows them to experience. Heroin further damages the amygdala. UCLA scientists think that long-term grief activates neurons in the reward centers of the brain, possibly giving these memories addiction-like properties. Brains may become rewired during severe stress and combat situations where soldiers experience almost nonstop violence and death. Their brains can establish alternate neural pathways that can be rewired after returning home with medical devices and acupuncture. Many of these soldiers become drug addicts when trying to self medicate to compensate for their altered brain reward system.

Quantum Brain Healing always considers substance abuse when treating PTSD and will attempt to remove harmful substances along with treating the PTSD. Many people suffering with PTSD also have a cigarette or tobacco addiction. Tobacco contains over four thousand chemicals; marijuana contains over four hundred chemicals. Tobacco increases dopamine levels and/or alters the nicotinic receptor sites in the brain. These receptor site problems can be treated successfully with NAET. All substance abuse, including cocaine, marijuana, heroin, alcohol, and nicotine, affects dopamine levels. These drugs activate the reward system and cause neurons to release large amounts of dopamine. Over time, dopamine overstimulates the brain to the point of damage, and higher levels of dopamine are needed to feel good. This altered neurotransmitter function impacts any activity that produces elevated moods. Drug abuse negatively impacts your sex life, your appetite, and your ability to feel pleasure or motivation for regular activities.

Methamphetamine decreases brain activity in about one year. There may be some parts of the brain that never recover from drug abuse. Abstinence combined with orthomolecular support during the neuron turnover period in the brain may completely repair the brain. This could be done with electro-acupuncture and brain stimulation. Up to 80 percent of PTSD patients are dually diagnosed with another psychiatric disorder, such as anxiety, major depression, substance abuse, cognitive impairment, memory loss, attention deficit disorder, or obsessive-compulsive disorder. Any rape victim, soldier in a battlefield, or person with a murder attempt made on his or her life has a very high chance of experiencing additional problems. PTSD has responded to increasing and stabilizing serotonin levels with antidepressants, amino acids, Bach Flower Remedies, and herbs.

The damaged amygdala can be repaired with an amino acid intervention that enhances the excitability of ITC cells to inhibit amygdala outputs. Functional imaging studies of the repair can help facilitate the optimal level of amino acids. This can be monitored with blood and urine tests. This could be partially accomplished with the opioid-blocking drug naloxone, but amino acids will work better, cost less, and create fewer side effects.

Diet

Many PTSD patients suffer with occasional or serious depression. The diet for PTSD patients suffering from depression should include fresh cold-water fish such as salmon and mackerel, eaten several times per week. Their diet should be high in unsaturated fats and may use snacks of walnuts and almonds. The cell membrane contains a small amount omega-3. Higher amounts of omega-3 levels could make a more stable and flexible cell membrane so that serotonin or dopamine remains in the cell longer. Purified fish oil may extend the life of serotonin, just as vitamin E and C can extend the life of other antioxidants. Fish oil has direct effects on neurotransmitter levels. This impacts bipolar disorder and depression prognoses. Other foods that are high in omega-3 essential fatty acids are also welcome for brain health.

Try to reduce or eliminate food additives, artificial sweeteners, high-fructose corn syrup, alcohol, nicotine, nitrates, refined foods, and food dyes. The diet should eliminate genetically modified foods and should include organic fruit and vegetables. A food-based multivitamin should be taken on a daily basis. One to two cups of Earl Gray tea per day may help many people with depression. It contains bergamot. Reduce your consumption of breads and pasta.

It is important for your daily protein level to be sufficient. Whey or rice protein can be taken for breakfast or as a snack food to increase your protein levels. People with depression may improve with a diet low in refined sugar. Stevia, molasses, maple syrup, and turbinado sugar are better choices for sweeteners.

Glutamate-Aspartate Restricted Diet (GARD)

The GARD is a type of elimination diet developed to treat epilepsy in animals that identifies foods and ingredients that should be avoided, including the following:

> gluten; commonly derived from wheat and grains

> casein; protein found in cow's milk (and most dairy products)

> soy

> corn, including corn syrup and corn derivative products

> MSG (monosodium glutamate); this a very common food ingredient in processed foods, even though it is rarely clearly labeled as such

> aspartame; commonly used as a sugar substitute

> glutamate; found in high concentrations in most beans/legumes

> hydrogenated oils

The GARD is a glutamate-aspartate restricted diet due to the limitation of these two nonessential, neurostimulating amino acids that are also the parent compounds of MSG and aspartame (NutraSweet). Aspartame is a neurotoxin which has been connected with brain cancer in Italy. Glutamate and aspartate are excitotoxins. They are able to trigger seizures and cause neurodegenerative diseases in some patients.

The GARD is also referred to as the gut absorption recovery diet due to its removal of gluten, dairy, soy, and corn. These foods may induce damage to the intestinal villi, resulting in celiac disease and food intolerance. This diet will work only if you avoid genetically modified foods.

Herbs for PTSD

Many single herbs for PTSD work wonders; you can find them online or at any local vitamin store. Be sure to purchase herbs that are not near their expiration date. Fresh herbs work best. You may be able to find seeds online and grow your own.

Milk thistle improves the immune system and reduces inflammation. It is an antioxidant. Quantum Brain Healing uses this herb to treat addiction withdrawal, eating disorders, anxiety, and depression. Eating disorders may be a result of an impaired liver function, where the liver and gallbladder are overactive. A well-functioning liver improves the outcome for many brain diseases. A healthy liver may result in less brain plaque.

Vinpocetine can be useful for many people in treating PTSD, ischemia, dementia, and memory loss. Vinpocetine may be useful in treating traumatic injury. This treatment would be best when tried within one to six months after the injury.

Lemon balm is used in Quantum Brain Healing to treat mania and other primary brain disease or secondary brain symptoms. Lemon balm is a sedative and antioxidant. It can be used to treat stress, anxiety, and nervous exhaustion caused by PTSD. Lemon balm is a great herb for its strong medical properties and mildness. It is an antiviral and antibiotic agent. It can act as an antidepressant for mild depression. Lemon balm acts on the hippocampus area of the brain and functions as an antispasmodic. It is an herb that can help prevent your hippocampus from shrinking. Lemon balm clears the brain for enhanced learning for those with a brain disease.

Catuaba is a South American herb that has many medical properties, including the ability to act as an antibiotic and antiviral. It also is an adaptogen that can sedate or stimulate the brain and central nervous system as needed. It is an antioxidant and may be an anti-aging herb. Catuaba sedates and calms the brain when overstimulated, as occurs from PTSD. This herb should be tried for two weeks, and if there is no improvement, it should be discontinued.

Skullcap can be used in addiction disorders for symptoms like withdrawal from barbiturates, alcohol, and tranquilizers. Skullcap can also treat problems such as headaches, neuralgia, hysteria, insomnia, anxiety, and other issues found in PTSD. This Quantum Brain herb should be used in an overall treatment plan for those suffering from addictions.

The flavonoids found in blueberries are called anthocyanins. They cross the blood-brain barrier to improve memory and affect the learning centers of the brain (including the hippocampus, cerebellum and cortex). This reduces brain inflammation and improves eyesight. It helps brain cells live longer, keeps the brain from forming brain plaque, and helps the brain make new brain cells. If you have experienced brain trauma, blueberry extract should be taken on a daily basis. If you want to avoid or delay Alzheimer's and Parkinson's, take this botanical flavonoid twice a day. It improves mood in some people due to its ability to increase dopamine.

Lobelia crosses the blood-brain barrier and increases norepinephrine release from the hippocampus. It stimulates the release of dopamine. It has a sedating affect and is an anxiolytic. It can increase cognitive performance. It may be useful in treating drug withdrawal symptoms, smoking cessation, depression, and headaches. It may also be useful in treating overall inflammation such as arthritic conditions. It helps with ADHD hyperactivity. It can help calm down symptoms of asthma.

Muira puama can stimulate or sedate, depending on what the person's body requires. It is an analgesic and reduces nerve pain. Muira puama is a neuroprotectant and extends the life of your brain cells and enhances memory. Muira puama can treat PTSD depression, stress, and anxiety. Do not take this herb without supervision.

Gotu kola indirectly impacts the level of certain neurotransmitters such as GABA, in the brain for cure and to treat depression and eating disorders. This herb directly affects the cortex of the brain. This herb can target the GABA receptor sites in the brain and balance neurotransmitter levels. Remember: any supplement taken to affect neurotransmitter levels must be supervised by your health care professional. This herb should not be taken by pregnant women or those trying to conceive a child.

Passionflower activates GABA receptors and sedates. It treats insomnia, anxiety, stress, neuralgia, headaches, delirium, and depression. Passionflower is an antibacterial, analgesic, and antispasmodic. It can increase circulation and lower blood pressure. Passionflower can be used as part of a strategy to treat nicotine addiction, alcoholism, and opiate withdrawal. Since addictions may become worse when people go extended periods of time without sleep, this herb can deal with both issues.

St. John's Wort may be used to treat insomnia and improve sleep quality. It is a sedative and an anxiolytic. It works in the brain to affect neurotransmitters by inhibiting the re-uptake of serotonin. It has been used to treat anxiety, stress, depression, phobias, seasonal affective disorder, obsessive-compulsive disorder, and post-traumatic stress disorder.

Start taking this herb immediately if you have PTSD. Astragalus can be used to treat brain symptoms associated the PTSD and is very inexpensive. Astragalus can improve brain issues connected with chronic fatigue, like brain fog. Astragalus can improve learning and increase memory. If the pituitary gland is impaired due to inflammation or viral attack, this herb could reverse the condition. Cancer and multiple sclerosis can be improved for many people using this herb due to its antiviral activity and its ability to enhance the immune system. It is an antiviral and antibacterial. It can help stomach problems due to extreme stress. Monitor your results.

217

Other herbs that help with PTSD include:

- ➢ Ginseng
- ➢ Rhodiola
- ➢ Horny goat weed
- ➢ Deer antler
- ➢ Black cohosh

Brain Stabilizing Supplements for PTSD and Brain Trauma

Melatonin is a hormone precursor and may be used in doses up to 3 mg per day and taken at night, thirty minutes prior to bedtime. This will help balance the brain and your circadian rhythm cycle to enhance your sleep. Melatonin will cross the blood-brain barrier and increase brain circulation. It strengthens the immune system. The enhanced immune system is due to the improvement in hormone and neurotransmitter regulation.

Vitamin C can be taken in large amounts to act as an antioxidant and detoxification agent. It will help your body fight stress and support your immune system. It is found in kiwi, oranges, lemons, cantaloupes, cherries, and many fruits.

Coenzyme Q10, or CoQ10, is an ubiquinone and a cofactor in the energy production. CoQ10 is best taken with food that contains some type of lipid or fat. This alleviates serious fatigue. Take this with 1500 mg per day malic acid for chronic fatigue syndrome or any extreme case of fatigue that is not due to viral or bacterial infection. It is important to get diagnostic testing for infections when extreme fatigue attacks and if you are suffering from depression. This should always be evaluated in situations of extreme fatigue, especially chronic. Undiagnosed sinus and lung infections may surface in this manner.

Choline is brain food. CDP-choline is a form of choline and cytidine. Choline is a precursor to phosphatidylcholine (PS). It is used in the structure and function of cells. It is a precursor to acetylcholine. CDP-choline can affect many neurological functions. Its actions include crossing blood-brain barrier. It improves immune and cognitive function for those with PTSD, as well as helping balance the brain—this action improves PTSD.

DHEA

DHEA is a natural hormone precursor to estrogen and androgen produced from cholesterol. Your body's own DHEA levels may be reduced by taking insulin, corticosteroids, opiates, or danazol. DHEA affects the brain in many ways, including improving mood. DHEA acts as an anti-inflammatory and immune enhancer.

The PTSD patient should include daily nutritional products to support achieving the best health possible in the least amount of time. The following list of supplements should be taken on a daily basis for those with PTSD:

- Lecithin
- Alpha lipoic acid
- B6
- B1
- Calcium, magnesium, and vitamin D supplement (combined)
- Life Extension Foundation multivitamin capsules
- Resveratrol

Orthomolecular Amino Acid Therapy

GABA is an amino acid that is a calming neurotransmitter; it is usually deficient in those with depression and anxiety. GABA may also be useful in treating OCD and insomnia.

5-HTP can calm overstimulated or overexcited nerves. This amino acid also can replace tricyclic antidepressants used in the treatment of neuropathy in some cases. 5-HTP may be used at higher doses to treat overeating related to mood disorders and depression.

Theanine is a great amino acid to treat those suffering from anxiety. It can relax and calm. It protects, balances, and extends the life of neurons. It may also prevent or delay the onset of four major brain diseases.

L-lysine acts like a partial serotonin receptor antagonist, inhibiting neurotransmitter re-uptake in the synapse. Lysine can reduce stress and chronic anxiety in people who have deficiencies of the amino acid.

DMG or dimethylglycine is a derivative of the amino acid glycine. It is also known as vitamin B-15 in Russia. In Russia, it is also used to treat drug addiction, alcoholism, autism, schizophrenia, children with minimal brain damage, senile dementia, and cognitive impairment.

Arginine is responsible for the secretion of hormones such as human growth hormone, glucagon, and insulin. It assists in wound healing, helps remove excess ammonia from the body, stimulates immune function, and promotes secretion of several hormones, including glucagon, insulin, and human growth hormone. It can be taken in IV form in extreme cases and can have impressive results. Take the arginine IV therapy after five of the Myers Cocktail IVs for impressive results.

Carnitine helps to access molecules from the body's fat stores to cells as energy to burn. It moves fatty acids through cellular membranes and cytosol into cells' mitochondria, where the fats undergo oxidation to produce ATP and increase cellular energy. Acetyl-Lcarnitine influences the regulation of the hormone pregnenolone produced by the adrenal gland. Pregnenolone deficiency is associated with low energy and extreme fatigue. Carnitine is found primarily from meat and dairy foods.

Acupuncture

Acupuncture is an ancient Chinese treatment to treat PTSD. It is usually combined with herbs. It is a holistic approach for treating and preventing disease. The main acupuncture tools are very thin needles, moxibustion, cupping, and electro-stimulation. Needles are inserted to points in the body. It modulates the limbic system, which provides a mechanism to treat mood disorders and addictions. Acupuncture can be used to treat many mood disorders and mental imbalances with an efficacy equal to pharmacology but without the side effects of drugs.

Acupuncture is effective in treating PTSD and is very good at calming the brain. PTSD causes extreme reactions, and acupuncture balances the brain to bring it into homeostasis. These problems can all be dramatically improved with acupuncture. The success of acupuncture arises from several factors, including patient compliance, diet, exercise, medical history, and practitioner expertise. At least thirteen sessions of acupuncture are recommended for PTSD; there should be significant improvement by the third treatment.

Electro-acupuncture can treat war injuries from gunfire and explosions by using six to thirteen needles in a circle the dragon fashion around a gun wound injury with scar tissue or gun shell fragments. The electro-acupuncture is done for thirty minutes and should be done four times before evaluating its success. This type of injury requires long term treatment and supplements that reduce inflammation in the body.

Electro-acupuncture also can reduce epileptiform discharges in the improved cognitive deficits and prevented shrinkage of areas within the limbic system of the brain. Electro-acupuncture functions as a neuroprotectant. It is likely that acupuncture and electro-acupuncture reverse signs of brain aging and mental decline.

Auricular acupuncture is often used to treat PTSD. The auricular points used for PTSD include shen men, blood pressure point, subcortex, brain, brain stem, cortex, kidney, mouth, and zero point. Several sessions will be required, and each session will take from thirty to forty minutes. Mourant acupuncture adds silver needles to this treatment, along with a sound meditation of violin or chanting from a monastery.

Scalp acupuncture treatments can also be used to treat PTSD. This is very good for motor injuries and sensory issues. The type of injury would not be the loss of a limb, rather the severe injury of a limb that remains functional. It could take several months of biweekly treatment in order to achieve the goal of full mobility. The scalp may be successful for the treatment of PTSD along with auricular acupuncture at the same time. Body points can also be used and include amnian, yin tang, stomach 25, heart 7, heart 9, small intestine 5, heart 3, lung 7, lung 3, urinary bladder 8, urinary bladder 20, urinary bladder 25, urinary bladder 63, urinary bladder 40, urinary bladder 27, pericardium 7, du 18, du 19, du 20, ren 1, ren 12, and ren 15.

Chinese Herbal Formulas

Several Chinese herbal formulas are used to treat PTSD; these are related to heat symptoms. The formulas would be chosen by symptoms and the root cause. The formulas are changed as the patient progresses. Ask an herbalist for guidance. There are at least twenty to forty formulas that may be useful for PTSD. The following formulas are for some of the more serious symptoms.

> **Bu Nao Wan,** Supplement the Brain Pills or Clear Mind from Kan

Traditional Chinese Medicine's therapeutic effects include tonifying heart yin, blood, and liver blood, transforming heart phlegm, calming the shen, nourishing the brain, strengthening the kidneys, and eliminating liver wind. Clear Mind is a Chinese herbal formula used to treat an overactive mind and enhance concentration or memory, mania, OCD, depression, anxiety, mental agitation, restlessness, fatigue, and insomnia.

> **Gun Tan Wan,** Vaporize Phlegm Pill or Chasing Away Phlegm Pill

TCM therapeutic effects include treating heat, phlegm-heat and phlegm-fire. Vaporize Phlegm Pill is a Chinese herbal formula used to treat acute mania; anxiety, neurosis;

221

dizziness, hysteria, nervous breakdown, heart palpitations, episodic mania, schizophrenia, bipolar disorder, tinnitus; acute bronchitis, agitated dreams, bizarre dreams, and coma.

> **Chai Hu Jia Long Gu Mu Li Tang** or Bupleurum D formula

TCM therapeutic effects include clearing heat from the liver and the heart, bringing down liver yang, sedating and calming the spirit, and unlocking the three yang stages. Bupleurum D formula is used to treat mania, rapid speech, emotional instability, irritability, restlessness, insomnia, hysteria, constipation, delirium, convulsions, and palpitations.

> **Bu Zhong Yi Qi Wan** or Supplement the Center and Boost the Qi Decoction

TCM therapeutic effects include tonifying qi, tonifying spleen qi, and lifting yang. Supplement the Center and Boost the Qi Decoction is a Chinese herbal formula used to treat anxiety, mania, various phobias, cerebral arteriosclerosis, dizziness, and stress.

> **Ding Xian Wan,** Stopping Epilepsy Pill; Arrest Seizures Pill; Gastrodia and Succinum Pill

TCM therapeutic effects include treating phlegm, wind, liver-wind, and opening the orifices. Arrest Seizures Pill is a Chinese herbal formula used to treat acute mania, dementia, nervous breakdown, bipolar disorder, clonic convulsion, infantile epilepsy, piercing scream, recurrent dizziness, alcohol and drug withdrawal, and dementia.

> **Huang Lian Jie Du Pian** or Coptis Relieve Toxicity

TCM therapeutic effects include treating heat from all three burners, blood heat, toxic heat, fire, damp heat, liver heat, and heart heat. Coptis Relieving Toxicity is a Chinese herbal formula used to treat mania, insomnia, bad breath, bleeding, delirium, palpitations, blood in stools or urine, incoherent speech, anxiety, emotional instability and dysentery.

> **Sheng Tie Luo Yin** or Iron Filings Decoction

TCM therapeutic effects include treating phlegm, phlegm-fire, calming the heart, calming the mind. Iron Filings Decoction is a Chinese herbal formula used to treat bad temper, extreme emotional instability, insomnia, irritability, mania, restlessness, aggressiveness, and screaming.

Emotional Freedom Technique (EFT)

Emotional Freedom Technique, or EFT, is a therapy that excels at treating pain or symptoms related to emotional thoughts, feelings, and trauma found in post-traumatic stress disorder (PTSD). Depression can be improved with EFT. This is a fairly inexpensive therapy that can be done with the help of a professional and reinforced by oneself at home. This therapy should be initially performed by an acupuncturist, chiropractor, Orthomolecular Medicine doctor, osteopath, or alternative medicine doctor.

EFT can benefit many people with disease and emotional trauma. It may alter the electromagnetic field of the patient. EFT uses fingers to perform a tapping motion on acupuncture points along energy meridians established in Traditional Chinese Medicine. This process is easy to perform on your own at home after a medical professional shows you the correct way to do the therapy. The points that are tapped on must be exactly correct in location. There may be additional points added to your treatment, depending upon your specific injury, disease, or level of emotional distress. This technique must usually be done more than once in order for it to succeed. Positive and negative affirmations are stated out loud while the tapping is done.

This therapy can alter your thoughts and feelings. Many diseases can improve and heal when the person changes her belief or thoughts concerning an illness or symptom. Many times, a patient's getting better can be as simple as getting someone to believe she can improve and helping her visualize this change in her life. Tapping may have this ability, along with moving the blocked energy along Chinese energy meridians. There are several energy meridians in the body, and they correspond to specific organs.

When the body's energy gets blocked or stuck in a specific organ, such as in the heart or small intestine, it may impact several organs and energy throughout the entire body. Chinese medicine believes that each energy meridian and organ is connected to emotions, directly or indirectly. As energetic blockages are removed and the energy flows freely, the person will improve the symptom and any emotionally caused problems can heal. It is possible for a person to get well in a single treatment. Many people will require several sessions. It can be used for healing depression, stress, anxiety, sleep disorders, migraines, seizures, and tics.

Eye Movement Desensitization and Reprocessing (EMDR)

EMDR helps treat emotional issues of all types, including PTSD, childhood trauma, automobile accidents, assault, natural disasters, sexual assault, personal failures, divorce, panic attacks, phobias, sexual addiction, computer or Nintendo addiction, and combat trauma. This is can be very effective for a person who has been gang-raped or assaulted by a gang or in a riot. EMDR may significantly help mania that has been triggered by an event rather than genetics. It could be massive stress tied to a nuclear meltdown at a power plant, radiation, earthquake, hurricane, tsunami, tornado, or landslide. The concept is a life-shaping event.

The doctor must initially analyze the patient's current situations, which trigger unemotional disturbance, and evaluate past traumatic events. Does the patient currently have the needed coping skills to prevent any similar circumstances from arising. If the patient has the skills, then the doctor may move forward.

A specific memory or event is identified and processed using EMDR procedures. The patient identifies the most specific image related to the memory and whatever negative feelings of self-worth are tied to this event. These feelings may include fear, nausea, headaches, crying, trauma, and inadequacy. The patient is given a positive image and belief to substitute for the problematic feeling or event. The intensity of the negative emotions should diminish during this treatment, and a positive emotion will root the patient.

The doctor helps the patient focus on the event and negative feeling, while body sensations are created. The patient moves his eyes rapidly and follows following the doctor's fingers as they move for approximately thirty to sixty seconds. The eye movements are used by all doctors; some doctors may add auditory sounds and tapping similar to Emotional Freedom Technique (EFT). The doctor asks the patient to describe the sensations that are being processed. This therapy can work wonders for people who experience massive amounts of fear, hysteria, mania, anger, and physical trauma. It may take four or five sessions of EMDR for this to resolve the issues of PTSD.

Biofeedback

Biofeedback may be used for psychological and stress problems. It can also be used to treat addiction issues. Many people suffer from chronic headaches, migraines, sexual dysfunction, mania, nervous stomach, essential hypertension, brain fog, anger management issues, and fear. These are classic symptoms of PTSD. This is a very good tool for PTSD and is often found at VA hospitals or psychologists' offices. Ask your doctor for biofeedback or neurofeedback; he may not think of it right away.

Biofeedback will improve most cases of PTSD. Chronic stress can cause some very serious problems. Chronic stress often leads to over-activation of the sympathetic nervous system. This is responsible for actions that are uncontrolled by conscious thought, such as blood pressure, hormones, increases in heart rate, and the constriction of blood vessels. The immune system fails under excessive long-term chronic stress, and symptoms and diseases surface.

Biofeedback machines can help people manage their bodies' reactions to reduce stress and related diseases. Insomnia caused by stress or anxiety can be resolved or improved. High blood pressure can be managed for some people with biofeedback. ADD, ADHD, anxiety, headaches, and migraines related to elevated blood pressure can fade. Addictions will be more easily dealt with and treated. Low-back pain can be treated with biofeedback. Teeth grinding and TMJ can improve with this therapy. It has also been used for seizure disorders and epilepsy of unknown origin. This may be used as a preventative to avoid or delay the onset of an autoimmune disease. It will take several sessions, and each session generally lasts about one hour. The sessions are moderately priced.

Hypnotherapy

Hypnotherapy can treat many disease symptoms associated with the brain. It can be used alone or in combination with other alternative medicine treatments. The National Institutes of Health (NIH) has approved hypnotherapy to treat chronic pain. Chronic pain, stress, anxiety, and migraines are often part of PTSD. Mayo Clinic's preliminary studies indicate that hypnotherapy can:

> Change negative behaviors, such as smoking, bed-wetting

> Binge eating, anorexia, and overeating

> Reduce or eliminate fears, stress, and anxiety

> Lower blood pressure (dizziness)

> Reduce the intensity or frequency of headaches, including migraines

Hypnosis will help many symptoms but not all, and it does not work on everyone. It requires patient motivation and a well-trained therapist. Hypnosis is a heightened state of concentration that creates a state of deep relaxation and quiets the mind. A hypnosis session is usually approximately one hour in length, and several sessions are needed for effective resolution. It may take three months of hypnotherapy to help someone with PTSD.

Hyperbaric Oxygen Therapy

In this type of therapy, patients breathe pure oxygen in a chamber with a higher-than-normal atmospheric pressure. This is reported to have successful results in treating some cases of epilepsy. This has been also used to treat carbon monoxide poisoning, viral-based pulmonary diseases, multiple sclerosis, dementia, cognitive impairment, stroke rehabilitation, and traumatic brain injury.

Intravenous Nutritional Therapy

The "Myers Cocktail" is an intravenous therapy consisting of mixing vitamins, minerals, amino acids, and other nutrients. It can be very useful in treating autoimmune diseases, chronic illness, viral infections, or digestive problems where oral nutrients are not being absorbed. When nutrients are given intravenously, your digestive system is bypassed and a much higher level of nutrition can be delivered directly to your cells via the bloodstream. Dr. John Myers was the first doctor to develop an intravenous nutrient therapy that obtained positive clinical results for a variety of medical conditions.

The Myers Cocktail IV therapy may be helpful for chronic or acute conditions, including PTSD, digestive problems, mental fatigue, fibromyalgia, depression, bacterial or viral infection, asthma, cardiac pain, congestive heart failure, palpitations, migraine headaches, cardiovascular disease, respiratory problems, seasonal allergies, hives, hyperthyroidism, and muscle spasms due to nutritional deficiency. PTSD resulting from extended trauma will be greatly helped with this therapy, particularly if there are significant dietary issues or mineral imbalances.

The Myers Cocktail improves the body's ability to make energy and increases cellular function. You may feel a warm sensation while the IV is administered. The effect is fast, but may take several treatments. It is administered by physicians or nurse practitioners.

Reflexology

Reflexology is based on the principle that the anatomy of the body is reflected in miniature reflex zones on the head, ears, hands, and feet. Reflexology promotes relaxation and reduces stress.

The reflexologist gently massages your feet and applies pressure to the reflexology points that correlate to your health problems. There are points that correlate to all the organs, glands, and body parts. In any disease, pressure is applied to the organs affected by the disease and the associated area of the disease. Reflexology areas correspond to the head, brain, brain stem, heart, lungs, kidney, gallbladder, pituitary, pineal/hypothalamus, thyroid, gonads, and adrenal glands areas.

Reflexology performed by an acupuncturist will include the use of the acupuncture points on the feet for a more complex and complete treatment. Some reflexologists apply pressure with their fingers, while others use small instruments. People with severe calluses or corns may be referred to a podiatrist for treatment prior to a reflexology treatment. Sessions typically last from thirty to sixty minutes. Acute diseases or trauma may be successfully treated in one or two visits, but chronic disease will require many treatments. Reflexology should be used for three to four months for PTSD, and the patient should ask for a copy of the map of points on the feet to massage on his own at home with lavender essential oils.

The nerve endings for the body are in the feet. Massage can calm the nervous system and relieve stress. Many reflexologists believe that manipulation of the feet reduces the lactic acid accumulation in the tissues and releases tiny calcium crystals that accumulate in the nerve endings of the feet. This restores the qi, or free flow of energy, from the feet to the corresponding organs. Other reflexologists believe that pressure on the reflex points may trigger the release of hormones, including endorphins—chemicals in the brain that naturally block pain. Reflexology creates relaxation, which improves circulation. Reflexology increases the body's rate of detoxification. Reflexology may be added monthly as an adjunct to more conventional therapy.

Bach Flower Remedies

Bach Flower Remedies originated as the work of Dr. Edward Bach and remain popular in many parts of the world today. The thirty-eight original flower essences developed by Dr. Bach have been the cornerstone of this field, which has expanded to Australian Bush Flower Essences and California Essences. Flower remedies are an integral part of holistic medicine.

All disease has a significant component that is driven by emotion. Flower essences may provide another manner of altering the energy of a disease, where desired brain function has not been achieved. A remedy captures the essence of the flower by harvesting at dawn during the height of the blooming season. The energetic field of the plant of flower is captured at its fullest in this manner. Flower essences alter a person's energetic field. I would consider this as a way to alter a stubborn case that had been not resolved with another therapy.

Listed below of some of the flower and plant essences and the emotions they may affect in some people:

- Agrimony; stress, concealed worry
- Aspen; apprehension anxiety
- Beech; intolerance, judgmental
- Centaury; passivity, weak willed
- Cerato; self-doubt
- Cherry plum; desperation, fear of losing self-control
- Chestnut bud; fails to learn by experience, absentminded
- Chicory; possessive, self-centeredness, self-pity

Music Therapy

Music therapy uses different instruments that impact the brain and body in specific ways. Your music therapist may not be trained specifically in treating PTSD, but there are many specific symptoms that can be relieved with music therapy, including depression, memory, sadness, concentration, anxiety, and stress. Music therapy has been clinically proven to be effective in managing and treating PTSD symptoms.

Hemi-Sync

Hemi-Sync involves binaural beating, a sensory-information stimulus, and changes the information sent to the reticular-thalamic activating system, which improves attention, focus, and level of awareness. Hemi-Sync signals contribute to a greater balance of the activity of the right and left hemispheres and cortical and subcortical areas of the brain. Hemi-Sync is used to improve PTSD, dyslexia, Asperger's, Down's syndrome, autism, learning disabilities, developmentally disabled, ADHD, OCD, brain trauma, bipolar disorder, cerebral palsy, seizure disorders, and to improve cognitive function in children with borderline IQ. You can purchase Hemi-Sync CDs for use at home on a regular basis. This system gets fairly good results.

The Tomatis Method (Listening Therapy)

Listening therapy is the method developed by Dr. Tomatis to treat conditions, including dyslexia, learning disabilities, ADHD, Down's syndrome, autism, depression, anxiety, behavioral problems, and chronic fatigue in both children and adults. This sound wave therapy was first developed in Europe in the 1950s, when Dr. Peter Manners developed a machine to heal with vibrations. A machine was placed on the afflicted area of the body and a frequency was matched to vibration of the cells of a healthy body. After treatment, the afflicted area resonated with healthy cellular frequency.

Dr. Manners developed a computerized system with about eight hundred frequencies that were used to treat a range of conditions. Similar therapies that pursue this concept are bio-resonance and vibrational therapy. Listening therapy is used to treat a wide range of diseases. It is not classically used to treat PTSD, but when the symptoms of PTSD include hysteria, ADHD, insomnia, and chronic fatigue, it could be tried and evaluated for several treatments. PTSD will benefit from this technique, and symptoms can diminish.

Yoga Enhancement with Heat and Herbs

Yoga is a great way to increase circulation, improve flexibility, reduce stress, balance hormone function, restore proper sleep cycles, and improve energy flow. There are many types of yoga and each offers different health benefits.

Power yoga is aerobic in nature and will burn more calories and improve circulation more quickly. It requires that the participant be healthy. A yoga posture, or asana, may be repeated quickly several times. There are standing and floor postures. Power yoga causes usually last one hour.

Hatha yoga increases balance, flexibility, and fitness at a gentle pace suitable for almost everyone. People of ages and levels of fitness can do this yoga. It is very important to discuss all health problems with the yoga instructor prior to class so you can be guided in which postures need to avoid for specific health concerns.

Bikram yoga, or hot yoga, is a great way to detoxify, increase flexibility, and increase metabolism. This practice involves performing yoga postures for ninety minutes in a heated room. The first half of the session involves standing postures, while the second half of the class is floor postures. Because muscles are warm, most people are able to increase flexibility at a faster rate. It is important to take water with you to class. Do not push yourself in this class until you are experienced in how the heat will affect you. Do not do this yoga every day, as it can result in electrolyte imbalances. If you are feeling dizzy after class, replenish your electrolytes with a supplement.

For some people with arthritis or other motion-limiting issues, herbs can improve their yoga practice. Herbs can increase flexibility, promote circulation, and stimulate the movement of energy. Herbs can aid in the proper performance of postures by improving circulation, joint function, balance, and coordination. They may be referred to as antirheumatic or anti-arthritic agents.

They are mainly herbs for Hatha yoga rather than to push the body during a yoga competition or for a power yoga class. Arthritis can benefit from taking herbs approximately 45 to 60 minutes prior to your class. Herbs that can be used in this fashion include adaptogenic herbs such as ashwagandha, panax ginseng, and huang qi. Other herbs used to improve circulation or flexibility in people with arthritis or motor-limiting issues include guggul, shallaki, myrrh, nirgundi, turmeric, saffron, curcumin, sage, salvia, Siberian ginseng, green tea, guarana, Bacopa monnieri, ginkgo biloba, angelica, kava kava, and dasha mula.

Several yoga poses are wonderful for helping balance the body to treat PTSD. These poses include Downward Facing Dog, Cat Pose, Child Pose, Easy Pose, Head to Knee Pose, Corpse Pose, and Fire Log Pose. Purchase an inexpensive yoga DVD, and do yoga in front of your TV screen to get the correct posture. Yoga is a fitness tool for a lifetime.

Qi Gong

Qi gong is an ancient type of Chinese energy work that improves health. It works on the prefrontal cortex and amygdala. It can heal anxiety, mild or moderate depression, and sleep disorders that are often found in PTSD. It increases brain relaxation and reduces the stress found in those with PTSD. It can increase your oxygen levels. It improves positive thoughts. PTSD has neurotransmitter imbalances that can re-balance with a daily Qi gong practice for 20 to 40 minutes per day.

Animal Therapy

Animal therapy includes horseback riding, swimming with dolphins, and helping train dogs. This therapy improves the coordination and motor skills of the patient, as well as the emotional well-being. Animals often are brought into VA hospitals or recovery facilities could help residents reduce stress and lower blood pressure. Dolphin therapy has been used for over thirty years. This could be an option for those suffering from PTSD in Hawaii and Florida. Children with PTSD may learn faster and retain information longer when they are with dolphins. Violent behavior associated with severe PTSD may be significantly reduced or eliminated. Animal therapy increases decision-making ability and self-confidence. Loss of control is a problem for many with PTSD and animal therapy can reestablish this concept for many. Most people have their stress levels reduced significantly by having a dog or cat. This is a form of unconditional love that is seldom found in daily life. PTSD patients can benefit from the responsibility of caring for an animal.

STRESS

Stress has a devastating impact on the brain. Uncontrollable stress is a major factor for brain disorders. Cellular changes in the hippocampus may lead to depression, post-traumatic stress disorders (PTSD), and Alzheimer's. Extended or repetitive stress affects memory and learning by affecting the part of the brain controlling and influencing cognitive function. Chronic stress may accelerate neurological structural changes, as well as cellular and molecular changes. Uncontrollable stress also leads to negative changes in the hypothalamus, pituitary, and adrenal system. Long-term stress can also permanently change the personality type.

Quantum Brain Healing relies on managing stress to prevent other health issues. Stress can go untreated and affect the brain in many serious ways. When stress is allowed go untreated, it progresses into depression, insomnia, anxiety, concentration issues, and memory problems. Stress negatively impacts the immune system. It can have huge impact on hormone and neurotransmitter levels. Stress is directly tied to cortisol levels. High cortisol levels are very dangerous and cause the body to gain weight without respect to diet.

Stress levels may also impact the prognosis of diabetes by altering the way your body handles glucose and raise overall glucose levels. Any bacterial infection gets worse with stress. You are less likely to take good care of yourself during times of high stress; you are more likely to have a poor diet and overeat. People often engage in recreational sex or drug use during high-stress periods. You can never anticipate how stress will impact every corner of your life. Viral infections may increase drastically. You may have less time to exercise. You may forget to take vitamins. You might drink too much caffeine. You might push yourself too hard.

Stress can be recognized by the many changes in your body, including pain, forgetfulness, memory loss, concentration problems, anger, changes in sleep patterns, fatigue, dietary changes, increases in consumption of alcohol and tobacco, eating disorders, and substance abuse. Stress can have many symptoms, including anger, fatigue, poor eating, poor work habits, stress eating, forgetting to eat, forgetfulness, insomnia, and increased levels of allergic reactions to foods. Some people may increase their time online with porn or gambling when suffering from increased stress.

Stress may be caused by job loss, bankruptcy, loss of a close friendship, betrayal of a husband or family member, home foreclosure, line of credit pull-back, physical injury, disease, car wreck, near-death experience, illness of a spouse of child, malnutrition, drug and alcohol abuse, emotional abuse, physical abuse, side effect of a medical drug, and failure to receive a promotion or raise. Poor relationships often increase stress levels at home at the office.

Often your timing can seriously impair relationships and increase stress. Discussing work problems outside the office may be a good idea. Move a troubling discussion to later in the day or another day to avoid stress. If a problem with a coworker occurs over breakfast or during a Monday morning staff meeting, reschedule interactions for later in the day. Each person has a biorhythm, and some times are better than others to interact with certain people. Limit stressful topics to a set amount of time, such as ten minutes.

Certain life events increase stress and anxiety, including major promotions, additional responsibility at work, remarriage, children, a new house, retirement, a death in the family, major illness, and layoffs.

Stressful events may require the addition of another amino acid, vitamins, minerals, or herb to handle this increased stress. Treating and healing stress with amino acids can reduce stress in the brain and repair its malfunction.

Many nutritional supplements have been used to relieve stress, and these should be used in addition to exercise and altering your routine. Incorporate any needed additional nutritional supplements into your diet so your body can handle stress better. Change your daily routine to include watching comedy shows or movies, working out at the gym, visiting an old friend, or having dinner at a favorite restaurant. Increase your fun time and reduce your exposure to problems at home and work until your stress level is reduced.

Stress often is reduced when there is adequate sleep and rest. You may need to invest in a new mattress if yours is older than twelve years old. New hypoallergenic pillows and sheets made from organic fabrics may be beneficial for some people. A ceiling fan may help a room with inadequate air flow. It may also be good to add an air ionizer. This can be found at the Sharper Image and is great for removing particles and dander from the air. It is also important for the air filter in the air conditioning system to be cleaned regularly or replaced. Clean any mold or fungus on the wall or in air conditioning with bleach.

Supplements that can help stress, including melatonin and a combination of calcium, magnesium, and vitamin D. It is extremely important to get the best-quality nutritional products. Eat yogurt, cottage cheese, milk, or dairy products to get calcium in your daily diet. Warm milk can be sipped at night before bed to help you sleep. Sex can also help people fall asleep. Avoid large quantities of alcohol when there is a sleep disorder. This impairs the brain-wave activity during the night.

Periods of extreme stress may increase the amount of the amino acids needed for a healthy brain. Quantum Brain Healing uses amino acid therapy for healing stress, including phenylalanine, L-tyrosine, L-lysine, L-tryptophan, 5-HTP, theanine, melatonin, and DHEA. Amino acid use is required for about three to six weeks before its success may be understood. It should be supported with vitamins and minerals in therapeutic amounts. Vitamin B and C supplements are always needed during times of severe stress. The body's metabolism uses far more of its vitamins during periods of extreme stress. Many people eat poorly during times of stress, which further deteriorates their health. Another good addition for people undergoing stress is a daily whole food-based multivitamin.

Orthomolecular Medicine uses theanine, SAM-e, and 5-HTP to help the body lower its levels of stress and anxiety. These amino acids should be taken on a daily basis for several months. They may be needed for several years for the body to balance. This concept addresses long-term job and marital stress that does not go away.

The requirement of certain vitamins increases during periods of extreme stress. Vitamin C requirements may increase by 200 percent during times of death or financial stress. Without the needed additional vitamins, your body may develop chronic fatigue or diabetes. Beta carotene requirements also increase, and sinus and skin infections may develop during periods of deficiency. Add CoQ10, alpha lipoid acid, vitamin C, B vitamins, zinc, selenium, folic acid, vitamin E, and chromium. Always take a food-based nutritional vitamin on a daily basis.

Myers Cocktail

The Myers Cocktail is an intravenous therapy consisting of mixing vitamins, minerals, amino acids, and other nutrients. It can be very useful in treating severe stress and autoimmune diseases, chronic illness, viral infections, or digestive problems where oral nutrients are not being absorbed. When nutrients are given intravenously, the digestive system is bypassed and a much higher level of nutrition can be delivered directly to your cells via the bloodstream.

The Myers Cocktail improves almost all digestive symptoms including bloating, diarrhea, food allergies, irritable bowel syndrome, colitis, ulcers, and Crohn's disease. It helps the body with fatigue and immediately increases energy levels. If your stress has depleted vitamins and minerals, this therapy can help deal with deficiency-related stress symptoms. Follow up this therapy with food-based vitamin supplements to extend the benefits.

The Myers Cocktail intravenous therapy improves the body's ability to make energy, and it increases cellular function. You may feel a warm sensation while the IV is administered.

Minerals

Quantum Brain Healing utilizes boron to treat stress. Without the proper minerals, your body will produce insufficient energy to produce optimal health. Boron is a trace mineral that functions as an activation agent and co-enzyme in your body's metabolism. This trace mineral helps regulate the levels of calcium, magnesium, and phosphorus.

You can find boron in apples, avocados, grapes, legumes, nuts, pears, plums, prunes, raisins, and tomatoes. Boron is an antioxidant and is a key anti-aging trace mineral. This most important use of boron in your body is to prevent and reduce inflammation. It also is important in helping the body fight viral infections by increasing the strength of the immune system.

Boron is involved in Quantum Brain Healing by its impact on hormone regulation. Boron affects estrogen and testosterone, which are key hormones in memory and cognitive thinking. It is involved in mental alertness, manual dexterity, hand-to-eye coordination, attention, perception, short-term memory, and long-term memory. Boron is very important in treating many brain diseases, like stress and cognitive impairment.

Quantum Brain Healing requires the addition of boron as a supplement. A high-quality supplement may be found in food-based vitamin and mineral products. Treating diseases with Orthomolecular Medicine usually requires higher levels of a substance than are found in most vitamin supplements or in foods. Diseases frequently increase the amount of a vitamin or mineral needed in the body to maintain good health. The RDA of vitamins and minerals is not sufficient for those suffering from serious illness or health issues.

Acupuncture

Acupuncture is an ancient Chinese treatment for stress and addiction. It is a holistic approach in treating and preventing disease. The main acupuncture tools are very thin needles, moxa, cupping, and electro-stimulation. Needles are inserted to points in the body. In Traditional Chinese Medicine, the acupuncture points, when needled, help balance the body's energy flow. Acupuncture can be used to treat stress and pain, generally or locally. It affects the cortex of the brain and the limbic system, which provides a mechanism to treat stress, mood disorders, and addictions without the side effects of drugs.

Acupuncture also is effective in treating Parkinson's, Alzheimer's, autism, anxiety, insomnia, mood swings, depression, poor memory, PTSD, ischemia, ADD, ADHD, OCD, mania, hemiplegia, seizures, dizziness, epilepsy, and addictions. Acupuncture is clearly able to alter the levels of neurotransmitters in the brain. Scalp, auricular, body, and laser acupuncture will improve and heal stress. Acupuncture can be used along with Chinese herbal formulas for very quick stress relief.

Bio-Identical Hormones

Bio-identical hormones may help treat and prevent stress if you are about age forty to fifty. Bio-identical progesterone may help balance the hormones for women in or nearing menopause. Men can also use androgen and testosterone bio-identical hormones to help them prevent memory loss and concentration issues. Amino acids, vitamins, and herbs are used in alternative medicine and Quantum Brain Healing to stimulate neurotransmitters to positively repair this damage.

Homeopathy

Homeopathy stimulates the body's defense mechanisms and processes so as to prevent or treat illness. It uses a diluted substance to treat a person. This dilution, or "remedy," would cause the illness or symptom if given at full strength.

Different homeopathic remedies treat stress or anxiety and are differentiated by symptoms. Focus on finding a knowledgeable practitioner. Discontinue taking the remedy if there has not been improvement after one month and/or seek another opinion.

Homeopathic products are for sale online and at various natural food stores, such as Whole Foods or Central Market. Some homeopathic practitioners custom-make remedies for each person.

The following homeopathic remedies may help with stress:

➢	Phosphoric ac.	for stress due to grief or bad news
➢	Picric ac.	for stress due to overwork
➢	Ignatia amara	for stress due to emotional upset. This may be related to losing a job, broken engagements, or the death of a spouse
➢	Nux	for stress due to overwork or excessive habits like overeating or excessive drinking or cigarette addiction

Aromatherapy

Aromatherapy is the controlled use of essential oil in treating stress, anxiety, brain disorders, bronchitis, depression, and other diseases. It may be utilized by itself or as an adjunct therapy along with other mainstream and alternative medical treatments. Its use dates back to biblical times. Traditional Chinese Medicine uses herbal remedies in an oil base that are very similar to essential oils in the treatment of arthritis, muscular strain, and back pain due to circulatory problems. Doctors in England are currently researching many different ways to use essential oils in a medical and healthcare setting.

Try lavender, lemon balm, bergamot, rose, and freesia essential oils for treating stress and anxiety. Be very careful not to use the essential oils directly on the skin without diluting them into a base oil, such as grape seed oil. Essential oils generally come in half-ounce and one ounce bottles. The essential oils will last longer if they are stored in dark blue or dark brown bottles.

Bach Flower Remedies

Bach Flower Remedies were invented by Dr. Edward Bach in England in the 1930s. The thirty-eight original flower essences developed by Dr. Bach have been the cornerstone in this field, which has expanded to Australian Bush Flower Essences and California Essences. Flower remedies are an integral part of holistic medicine. A remedy captures the essence of the flower when it is harvested at dawn during the height of the bloom season. The energetic field of the plant is captured at its peak.

All disease has a significant component that is driven by emotion. Flower essences may provide another manner of altering the energy of a disease where desired brain function has not been achieved. Flower essences definitely alter the energetic field of a person. Flower and plant essences heal the emotions in some people. The plant essence of agrimony treats stress.

Glandular Supplements

The use of glandular supplements must be supervised by a doctor or acupuncturist. Adrenal supplements may be great for people whose adrenal glands are not functioning at normal levels. Thyroid glandular supplement is another great option for those with an underachieving thyroid or a number of chronic bacterial infections. Many people suffering from chronic sinus infections can cure the issue with thyroid medication or thyroid glandular supplements. Armour thyroid is an example of a glandular thyroid medicine.

Thymus glandular supplements may help some people with immune deficiency problems. The

T-cell count should be about four hundred before you incorporate this glandular supplement. These supplements must be organic. Glandular supplements can be either porcine or bovine. Jewish or Muslim people may want to avoid porcine supplements. They should look for organic bovine supplements. Enzymatic Therapy and Standard Process are good brands and are well manufactured.

Herbs

Lemon balm is a sedative and antioxidant. It can be used to treat stress and anxiety. Its sedative effect can benefit nervous exhaustion or reduce signs of aging. Aging of the brain may be accelerated by bacterial and viral infections. Any herb that has antibiotic and antiviral actions may be taken on a regular basis to prevent this type of occurrence. Green tea falls into this category.

Lemon balm is an acetylcholinesterase inhibitor and can help Alzheimer's and Parkinson's in their earliest phases by delaying the onset. It can be used to prevent mild to moderate dementia. Lemon balm inhibits the production of the thyroid hormone and could help treat Hashimoto's disease in its early phase. It can also treat hyperthyroid or Graves' disease. Do not take this herb if you have hypothyroid disease or take thyroid medicine. Lemon balm acts on the hippocampus area of the brain and functions as an antispasmodic. It can treat ADHD hyperactivity and migraine headaches. Lemon balm can help clear the brain for enhanced learning for those with a brain disease.

Quantum Brain Healing uses vitamins, minerals, amino acids, nutritional supplements, and herbs in high doses to treat and heal brain disease. These supplements may be combined with other therapies. There may a focus on removing the toxins before adding in the supplements. Chinese club moss is a very important herb that is used for many of the most serious brain illnesses.

Chinese club moss can increase energy levels, strengthen the immune system, increase alertness, improve learning, increase memory, impact neurotransmitter levels, and improve nerve function by strengthening and lengthening the nerve impulse. It can act as a brain enhancer.

Chinese club moss is beneficial for many diseases and conditions, including Alzheimer's, myasthenia gravis, Parkinson's disease, memory loss, dementia, and cognitive impairment. Chinese club moss may be useful in reducing symptoms of Huntington's disease, multiple sclerosis, and spastic symptoms of undiagnosed diseases.

Chinese club moss must be combined with a good diet and large quantities of vitamins and minerals. With stress, the RDA is insufficient to improve the condition. Very large doses of vitamins are needed to achieve the best outcome. It is likely that once the body has a major disease, the level of vitamins and minerals needed for basic metabolism is increased. A major detoxification should be implemented early for all diseases. Research is very inconclusive, but many theories suggest that toxic pesticides and chemicals are at the root of diseases like Alzheimer's, cognitive impairment, early dementia, and unexplained memory loss.

Horny goat weed can reduce stress due to low neurotransmitter levels. It increases levels of epinephrine, norepinephrine, serotonin, dopamine, and testosterone. It may also increase thyroid levels, if they are suboptimal. Horny goat weed reduces cortisol levels in the body during periods of high stress. It also reduces abnormal cellular glucose levels. High glucose levels cause inflammation, accelerate aging, reduce libido, and lower sexual performance.

Quantum Brain Healing uses kava to sedate the overactive brain; this can treat stress. Kava acts on the limbic system, and it affects several neurotransmitters, including GABA and noradrenaline. The limbic area of the brain is instrumental to emotions of sadness, fear, and anger. It may be an adaptogen due to its slight ability to elevate mood and sedate.

Frequently, herbs can produce two opposing actions, depending upon what is needed by the body—these are considered adaptogens. Taking kava is associated with lower levels of leukemia and ovarian cancer, according to a study at the University of Aberdeen in Scotland. It is important to note that there are reports of severe liver toxicity by a few on kava. This may be due to problems with how kava is made or other substances that the patients are consuming while on this herb.

Kava can be used to treat anxiety, nervousness, stress, and insomnia. These conditions are related for many people, and the slight sedating effect that kava has may resolve anxiety and stress. Kava also treats agoraphobia and may be tied to its ability to affect the limbic area of the brain.

Kava must be supported with vitamins, minerals, and high levels of antioxidants. A break should be taken from this herb on a regular basis. Eat a wide variety of organic vegetables and fruits while taking kava. Avoid alcohol, cigarettes, nicotine, and recreational drugs when taking kava. Do not do anything to overload the liver. A regular liver detoxification is a good idea for anyone taking kava.

This is not recommended for those with Parkinson's, liver disease, lung disease, depression, or bipolar disorder. Kava has negative interactions with acetazolamide, amiloride, furosemide, or with angiotensin-converting enzyme (ACE) inhibitors such as benazepril, captopril, lisinopril, quinapril, ramipril, levodopa-based medication, alcohol, Xanax, barbiturates, or other mood-altering drugs.

Many diseases are improved with hawthorn, including stress, ADHD, memory loss, arteriosclerosis, ischemia, stroke, and Alzheimer's. Hawthorn is a small berry that is commonly used to treat heart conditions and has been used for centuries. Hawthorn is also used to several serious brain diseases. This herb can be taken as a tea or a capsule supplement. If there is heart disease, a food-based vitamin and CoQ10 supplement should be added on a daily basis. The Quantum Brain Therapy uses hawthorn and several amino acids to impact the brain's circulation, oxygenation levels, and any inflammation.

Hawthorn can cross the blood-brain barrier and affect the brain directly; for example by increasing blood circulation, lowering blood pressure, decreasing cholesterol, and acting as an antibiotic, anti-inflammatory, and antioxidant.

It is possible that many brain diseases begin when there are heart problems the damaged heart's failure to properly oxygenate the brain can cause many problems. A heart condition leads to poor circulation, which may increase the amyloid protein buildup in the brain. The other possibility is that impaired circulation increases stress, and the increased stress causes the other brain diseases to manifest.

Emotional Freedom Technique (EFT)

When the body's energy gets blocked or stuck in a specific organ, it may impact several organs and energy throughout the entire body. As energetic blockages are removed and the energy flows freely, the person will improve and any emotionally caused problems can heal. Chinese medicine believes that each energy meridian and organ is connected to emotions, directly or indirectly. It is possible for a person to get well in a single treatment, but many people will require several sessions. EFT helps in treating stress, anxiety, addictions, and eating disorders.

This is a fairly inexpensive therapy can be done with the help of a professional and reinforced by oneself at home. This therapy should be initially performed by an acupuncturist, chiropractor, Orthomolecular Medicine doctor, osteopath, or alternative medicine doctor.

EFT uses fingers to perform a tapping motion on acupuncture points along energy meridians established in Traditional Chinese Medicine. The points that are tapped on must be exactly correct in location. There may be additional points added to your treatment, depending upon your specific injury, disease, or level of emotional distress. This technique must usually be done more than once in order for it to succeed. Positive and negative affirmations are stated out loud while the tapping is done.

This therapy can alter your thought and feelings. Many diseases can improve and heal when the person changes her belief or thoughts concerning an illness or symptom. Many times, a patient's getting better can be as simple as getting someone to believe she can improve and helping her visualize this change in her life. Tapping may have this ability, along with moving the blocked energy along Chinese energy meridians.

EFT has not been extensively studied or published, and there have not been adequate double-blind studies on this therapy in America.

Bio-Mat

The Bio-Mat is a device that uses far infrared and amethyst crystals. The patient lies on the mat for twenty or thirty minutes and listens through earphones to sounds and instructions. It seems like a meditation session, and it relaxes your body as the infrared speeds the elimination of toxins. It also ionizes your body with negative ions, which improves your body's ability to heal. This should normally be used about twice a week on the depression patient. The Bio-Mat, however, is not inexpensive—it can cost upwards of $2,500, depending on the size you choose—but it is a unique device. It is a patented device, and there is one manufacturer. The increase in your body's ability to expel toxins will reduce the toxic load on your liver. This may be one of the ways it reduces stress. Another possibility is that negative ions help people feel better.

Biofeedback

Biofeedback may be used for psychological and stress problems. It can also be used to treat addiction issues. Many people suffer from chronic headaches, migraines, sexual dysfunction, migraines, nervous stomach, essential hypertension, RSI, brain fog, anger management issues, tics, and neuropathy. Multiple therapies may be needed, and this is a good tool. Biofeedback may be better for some people who have diseases that are rooted in stress.

Chronic stress can cause serious problems. It often leads to over-activation of the sympathetic nervous system. This is responsible for our actions that are uncontrolled by conscious thought, such as blood pressure, hormones, increases in heart rate, and the constriction of blood vessels. The body works to achieve a balanced state, and when it is unable to do so, it causes stress-related disease. The immune system fails under excessive,

240

long-term chronic stress, and symptoms and diseases surface.

Biofeedback machines can help people manage their bodies' reactions to reduce stress related diseases. High blood pressure can be managed for some people with biofeedback. It will take several sessions, and each session generally lasts about one hour. The sessions are moderately priced.

Hypnotherapy

Hypnotherapy can treat many disease symptoms associated with the brain. It can be used alone or in combination with other alternative medicine treatments. Mayo Clinic's studies indicate that hypnotherapy can:

> change negative behaviors, such as smoking, bed-wetting

> binge eating, anorexia, and overeating

> reduce or eliminate fears, stress, and anxiety

> lower blood pressure (dizziness)

> reduce the intensity or frequency of headaches, including migraines

Hypnosis will help many symptoms but not all, and it does not work on everyone. It requires patient motivation and a well-trained therapist. Hypnosis is a heightened state of concentration that creates a state of deep relaxation and quiets the mind. A hypnosis session is usually approximately one hour in length, and several sessions are needed. It may require follow-up treatments for severe continued stress, such as that caused by death of a loved one or marital disasters like divorce.

Exercise

Exercise is a cure for treating stress, mild anxiety, and moderate depression. The exercise can be yoga, tai chi, qi gong, ballet, golf, biking, hiking, or walking, dancing, or gardening. People with depression should be outside and exposed to sunlight at least thirty minutes per day.

Exercise to reduce stress should be done at least four days per week, unless there is an injury that prevents it. People who regularly engage in exercise or meditation show far less stress in their bodies. Their bodies age more slowly, and they experience less disease.

Yoga

Hatha yoga increases balance, flexibility, and fitness at a gentle pace suitable for almost everyone. People of ages and levels of fitness can do this yoga. It is very important to discuss all health problems with the yoga instructor prior to class so you can be guided in which postures you need to avoid for specific health concerns. Yoga is a great way to increase circulation, reduce stress, balance hormone function, restore proper sleep cycles, and improve energy flow.

Herbs intended for Hatha yoga enhance the yoga practice. These herbs include adaptogenic herbs such as ashwagandha, panax ginseng, and huang qi. Other herbs used to improve circulation or flexibility in people with arthritis or motor-limiting issues include guggul, shallaki, myrrh, nirgundi, turmeric, saffron, curcumin, sage, salvia, Siberian ginseng, green tea, guarana, Bacopa monnieri, ginkgo biloba, angelica, kava kava, and dasha mula.

Power yoga is aerobic in nature and will burn more calories and improve circulation more quickly than other types. It requires that the participant be healthy. The power yoga class has standing and floor postures, and the class usually lasts one hour.

Bikram yoga, or hot yoga, is a great way to detoxify, increase flexibility, and increase metabolism. This practice involves performing yoga postures for ninety minutes in a heated room. The first half of the session involves standing postures, while the second half of the class is floor postures. Because muscles are warm, most people are able to increase flexibility at a faster rate. It is important to take water with you to class. Do not push yourself in this class until you are experienced in how the heat will affect you. Do not do this yoga every day, as it can result in electrolyte imbalances. If you are feeling dizzy after class, replenish your electrolytes with a supplement. Avoid Bikram yoga if you know or suspect that you have MS or any autoimmune disease. Diseases that debilitate you and weaken you can make you more vulnerable to overheating when exposed to extreme heat. This can lead to heat stroke. Poor hydration can negatively impact this issue.

Animal Play Therapy

Animal therapy has helped children who have brain dysfunction. Animal therapy includes horseback riding, swimming with dolphins, and helping train dogs. This therapy improves the coordination and motor skills of the patient, as well as the emotional well-being. Animals are being brought into retirement homes because of their ability to help residents reduce stress and lower blood pressure. Dolphin therapy has been used for over thirty years. Most people have their stress levels reduced significantly by having a dog or cat. This is a form of unconditional love that is seldom found in daily life.

Increasing Brain Function

Quantum Brain Healing finds many ways to stimulate brain function and increase intelligence, including increasing the number of sensory inputs, changing and improving the body with nutrition and supplements, adjusting physical environment, and creating a supportive environment. Anything that increases blood flow to the brain or increases mental activity is capable of increasing intelligence, memory, or concentration. The addition of Chinese medicine and acupuncture is an important way to add neural pathways to the brain and enhance brain repair. The ability to increase your brain function is directly tied to reduction of stress levels for many people.

Brain circulation can be increased by using herbs, acupuncture, music therapy, Hemi-Sync Technology, nutritional supplements, nootrophics, deep breathing, yoga, Zen meditation, physical exercise, brain exercises, researching on the Internet, card games like bridge and blackjack, and crossword puzzles. Memory also be can improved by detoxifying heavy metals and chemicals with far infrared sauna, hot yoga, sweat-producing exercise, foot ionizing detox, and detoxification diets.

Quantum Brain Healing believes that any substance that encourages the formation of new neurons or new neural pathways will increase brain speed, increase available functioning brain tissue, or prevent neuron loss. It can alter the neural pathways connecting the brain hemispheres. This gives the brain more options.

It has been recently discovered that humans emit photons of light from many areas of the body, including the forehead. This new area of science has been researched in the United States, Japan, and China. It has not yet been determined if there is a correlation between photon levels and brain disease. A base level would need to established and monitored when disease occurred. Another interesting experiment would be to see if there is a correlation between intelligence and spiritual levels, emotional types, and photons.

Recent research in sound therapy has looked at increasing the ability of the ear and brain in handling higher frequency than is normal. This can affect learning, memory, and concentration. Another way to improve math, memory, concentration and learning ability from 100 to 600 percent is a program called Speed Learning. This would be a great addition for any family with young children or for older people re-entering college. It could also be used by the army and marines for veterans retuning from battle with head injury or trauma.

Fluid intelligence is the ability to solve problems or issues by establishing relationships

243

between concepts or ideas where there may have been no previous relationship, knowledge, or skills. Fluid intelligence is used in many cognitive tasks, learning, and professional and educational success. Traditional cognitive training does not have a high correlation with fluid intelligence. It is now possible to increase fluid intelligence through intense memory work or memory training. Fluid intelligence increases with amount of total time of memory training or work- this includes Internet and library research. It is unknown exactly how much memory training or exercise may be required for lasting effects.

There are a number of new software programs available to achieve fluid intelligence in a cost-effective manner. There are also many types of music and sound therapy that improve fluid intelligence. Listening to many types of music and switching the type of music frequently on several times a day on a daily basis allows new neural pathways to form, and this increases intelligence. Listening to rock or jazz music in the morning and classical music in the evening is a good example of this concept. Switching any routine on a frequent basis in everyday life will increase the number of neural pathways formed.

Emotional blockage can impair brain focus and ability to function. Bach Flower Remedies can be used successfully to reduce and dissipate emotional trauma, stress, and blockages. As the emotions are processed, the brain will perform at a higher level.

There is a concept that spending your time with creative, brilliant people will increase your intelligence. This is difficult to prove because any group of brilliant people would be different, but this is similar to the concept of playing tennis with a better player in order to improve your game. This concept is very evident in the music world, chess, bridge, master painting classes, and any competitive sport.

Diagnosis and treatment of hormone deficiencies can create impaired memory and concentration problems, especially for thyroid, estrogen, or testosterone hormones. Food allergies can create many mind problems. Sugar creates much inflammation, and other commonly eaten foods will create problems in short and long-term memory, concentration, spatial arrangement, and repetitive-pattern learning. NAET, rotation diet, elimination diet, and the brown rice cleanse can successfully treat food allergies. A diet extremely high in organic vegetables and fruits will reduce oxidation levels and reduce the production of free radicals throughout the body.

Dietary changes should occur and should include an initial detoxification of all heavy metals and pesticides. It is possible for heavy metals and pesticides to induce Alzheimer's or Alzheimer's like symptoms from serious toxin overload. Detoxification can be done with oral chelators and a pure diet. Vitamins, minerals, and orthomolecular amino acid therapy can enhance mental function, improve memory, and increase motor coordination. Bio-identical hormone replacement therapy can be used to improve energy, concentration, and memory.

People who want to increase their IQ should reduce stress, get adequate sleep, stay hydrated, eat regular meals, and have an organized routine. Try to delegate unimportant work or tasks to others. Keep your work day organized with large blocks of time for your work without interruption. Put your phone on hold, and let the calls role into voice mail. It may help to leave the office during the day for a brief walk. Use your company gym or workout facilities. Try to sneak a yoga class into your lunch hour twice a week. Keep busy with mental activities like learning a second language, Internet games, playing cards, or playing bridge. Dominos, chess, backgammon, or large, complicated puzzles will also improve brain function.

Yoga and qi gong are wonderful ways to balance hormones and neurotransmitters and increase cellular energy production. Higher brain function requires a higher level of available energy produced on a cellular level and more available neuro-supporting supplements. Orthomolecular Medicine can introduce amino acids like SAM-e, carnitine, orthinine, and arginine to increase energy production, cardiac function, and increase metabolism rates.

Porcine or bovine thyroid glandular supplements can be used to improve memory, concentration, and intelligence in people with low or borderline thyroid levels. Porcine glandular supplements are closer to human chemistry than bovine. Deficiency symptoms include hair loss, constipation, weight gain, susceptibility to infections and illness, brittle nails, depression, memory lapses, concentration problems, irritability, fatigue, low energy, dry or cracked skin, cold intolerance, anxiety, thinning of the outer eyebrows, excessive sleep, low body temperature, low sex drive, and menstrual problems. Successful supplementation should be carefully monitored with frequent basal temperature monitoring or blood tests. Supplements from animals raised on organic or chemical-free farms are best.

Long-term deficiency of omega-3 and omega-6 fatty acids can seriously impair concentration, learning, memory, and neural plasticity. Neurotransmitter and amino acid deficiencies will also result in impaired memory and intelligence.

Drinking pure water is a good idea, as dehydration is one of the chief ways that brains become sluggish. Alcohol is able to destroy brain cells and should be avoided in excess. Foods that are extremely high in antioxidants are good neuroprotectants. The following foods can enhance the brain by increasing clarity, memory, and intelligence:

- Açai berry extract
- Blueberries

- ➢ Blackberries
- ➢ Raspberries
- ➢ Cherries
- ➢ Prunes
- ➢ Strawberries
- ➢ Raisins
- ➢ Red grapes
- ➢ Plums
- ➢ Kale
- ➢ Spinach
- ➢ Brussels sprouts
- ➢ Walnuts
- ➢ Almonds
- ➢ Flaxseed
- ➢ Cold-water fish
- ➢ Coffee
- ➢ Tea

There are many brain-enhancing herbs to improve memory and concentration, reverse neuron loss, decrease brain fog, increase the transfer of information between the brain hemispheres, sharpen mental focus, prevent memory loss, calm an overactive brain, and increase intelligence. These herbs can be combined with cofactors to speed their action in the body. They can be used alone or in combination and should be examined for their potentiation effects on one another. These can be combined with medical devices to stimulate the brain and enhance their effects.

Herbs

The herbs found below can help increase IQ or improve the performance of the brain:

- ➢ Muira puama

Muira puama crosses blood-brain barrier. It increases circulation in several areas of the brain, including the hippocampus, cerebral cortex, hypothalamus, and cerebellum and the central nervous system. It protects memory and is an antioxidant. The herb may have use in treating impaired nerve function due to accident or trauma. Muira puama is an adaptogen and can stimulate or sedate, depending on what the person's body requires. It can stimulate the immune system. It is an analgesic and reduces nerve pain. The analgesic mechanism can affect the central nervous system and reduce inflammation and swelling. Muira puama is a neuroprotectant and extends the life of brain cells.

> ## Vitex

Vitex (chasteberry or Agnus castus) increases prolactin levels. Vitex is an adaptogenic herb that can balance hormones and increase or decrease the level of prolactin. If you have low prolactin, supplementation can assist the anterior lobe of the pituitary gland to increase production of prolactin. Increasing levels of prolactin and vasopressin will increase the neural stem cells, which results in an increased level of brain cells. Increases in brain cells and neural pathways can translate into increased IQ. The best way to facilitate this is to take other substances that target the hippocampus and increase neural plasticity. This combination could increase the IQ by approximately 12 percent.

> ## Brahmi

Brahmi is an Ayurvedic herb that improves protein synthesis in brain cell repair and encourages new neuron growth. Implementing acupuncture with herbs and amino acids to stimulate new nerve growth is suggested. The acupuncture will help facilitate new neural networks. The acupuncture may work more quickly if electro-acupuncture is used.

> ## Gotu Kola

Gotu kola indirectly impacts the level of certain neurotransmitters levels like GABA in the brain to cure and treat depression and eating disorders. This herb directly affects the cortex of the brain. This herb can target the GABA receptor sites in the brain and balance neurotransmitter levels. This herb may slow brain aging and delay the death of brain cells. It can delay dementia and prevent memory loss. Remember that any supplement taken to affect neurotransmitter levels must be supervised by your health care professional. This herb should not be taken by pregnant women or those trying to conceive a child.

> ## Chinese Club Moss

Chinese club moss must be taken with vitamins and minerals. It can increase energy levels, strengthen the immune system, increase alertness, improve learning, increase memory, impact neurotransmitter levels, and improve nerve function by strengthening and lengthening the nerve impulse. It can act as a brain enhancer.

> ### Piracetam

Piracetam acts by increasing brain circulation, increasing cholinergic receptors in the brain, enhancing memory, and acting as a neuroprotectant. It enhances the functioning of the right temporal lobe. It prevents stress, anxiety, and depression, and improves the memory. All these functions improve brain function and IQ.

> ### Vinpocetine

Vinpocetine is a periwinkle extract that crosses blood-brain barrier and acts as a neuroprotectant for brain cells and keeps them alive longer. Vinpocetine is an antioxidant that improves brain circulation and metabolism. It reduces stress and memory loss. It increases brain metabolism. It is an effective long-term brain enhancer and can reduce brain fog and help with learning and concentration problems to increase IQ. It is best when combined with yoga or tai chi for increased brain circulation.

> ### Lemon Balm

Lemon balm is a sedative and antioxidant that acts on the hippocampus area of the brain. It can be used to treat stress and anxiety. Its sedative effect can benefit nervous exhaustion. Lemon balm also acts on the brain in many ways to reduce signs of aging. Aging of the brain may be accelerated by bacterial and viral infections that go undiagnosed and untreated. Any herb that has antibiotic and antiviral actions may be taken on a regular basis. An overactive brain can increase its mental focus and concentration with this herb. It can also improve mental clarity.

> ### Ginseng

Ginseng, an adaptogen that increases the amount of energy made by the brain cells, improves short-term memory and concentration. It is an antioxidant and neuroprotectant. This herb reduces brain inflammation, which can help brain fog and learning. It can increase the brain's ability to grow new cells, and this delays aging. It can be used for improving cognitive disorders like retention and access to information. Ginseng can increase IQ in those with lower IQ levels when taken on a long term basis in combination with scalp acupuncture and electro-acupuncture. It lowers glucose levels in the cell this may be due to an increase in energy production of the mitochondria. It helps the brain fight disease due to its ability to function as an immune enhancer.

> ### Ginkgo Biloba

Gingko crosses the blood-brain barrier and regulates the tone and elasticity of blood vessels. It protects and regenerates neurons. Brain cells can last longer when exposed to this herb. It is an antioxidant and is anti-aging. This herb can reduce brain age by years when taken on a long-term basis. This herb can help older people with balance issues and those suffering from vertigo. It prevents senile dementia and memory loss. It slows the growth of brain tumors. Take this in very large quantities in combination with two other herbs for the maximum anti-aging effect.

Gingko is beneficial for teenagers and college students with poor concentration. It treats cognitive disorders. It can prevent headaches and treat migraine by increasing blood flow and circulation. It can prevent depression and is a memory enhancer for aging patients. Leukemia patients who take ginkgo when their disease is in remission may reverse brain damage that may occur from the disease and treatment; they should also take astragalus for several months. Do not take ginkgo with blood thinners. Monitor this herb very carefully for the best results.

> ### Himalayan Rhodiola Sacra

Rhodiola is an adaptogenic herb that can balance your brain. It is an antioxidant and reduces free radicals in your brain. This slows brain aging and supports brain cells. It increases energy production of ATP produced by the mitochondria in your brain cells. It can also increase production and circulation time of neurotransmitters in the brain. Rhodiola increases learning and sharpens focus and memory. It increases the permeability of the brain cells to serotonin and dopamine to their receptor sites. It allows the brain to adapt to stress and anxiety. It improves depression and reverses some cases of insomnia when the herb from the Himalayas. The Rhodiola herb found in Siberia, however, is stronger and can cause insomnia; it is closer to ginseng in its ability to stimulate the body.

> ### Skullcap

Skullcap is used for calming or sedating a part of the brain. Anxiety, stress, mania, hyperthyroid, MS, ALS, memory loss due to physical or emotional trauma, anger, or inflammation all can be helped with skullcap. These issues can slow learning, impede memory, impair concentration, and interfere with spatial arrangement skills. This herb can help restore IQ that has been impaired from excess brain inflammation and over stimulation. It can balance neurotransmitter levels and is anti-convulsive and anti-inflammatory. It can help repair IQ problems that were rooted in alcoholism and drug abuse. Skullcap can benefit teenagers whose brains have been negatively impacted with drugs or alcohol. (It will not work it the substance abuse has not been eliminated.)

> ### Jamaican Dogwood

Dogwood is an analgesic and can reduce inflammation in an overstimulated brain cell or nerve cell. It is an antispasmodic and antitussive herb that has sedative properties. Dogwood can reduce fear and anxiety. It is beneficial for extreme trauma or fear-based issues. This herb has a strong analgesic property that rivals those found in drugs. It treats neuralgia, memory loss, neuropathy, insomnia, and migraine headaches. Jamaican dogwood may be combined with lemon balm to effectively treat pain of migraine headaches. This is a great herb to add to other herbs for managing over stimulation and inflammation.

> ### Sage

Sage is an herb that reduces stress and anxiety. It acts like mild estrogen in the brain and improves memory and concentration. It is anti-inflammatory, antioxidant, anti-fungal, and antibiotic. This herb is an anti-aging herb for the brain. It inhibits acetylcholine and acts on the central nervous system. This is not the best choice for those with low serotonin or dopamine levels. It could help those with Alzheimer's or MS. It slows and helps prevent memory loss.

> ### Bacopa monnieri

Bacopa is an Indian herb that is a neuroprotectant and is amazing in its ability to mildly sedate the brain; it can replace the pharmaceutical Vicodin. It increases memory capacity and motor learning ability and improves speed of visual information processing. It reduces beta-amyloid deposits in the brain. It can reduce inflammation and anxiety. Bacopa monnieri can be used to help those with dyslexia. It is the fifth most important herb in anti-aging medicine for the brain. You can find out more about this herb in the literature available at the American Academy of Anti-Aging Medicine and Life Extension Foundation.

> ### Ashwagandha

Ashwagandha is a brain and immunity enhancer. It can improve memory. It inhibits inflammation and fights tumor formation. It has an ability to interact with the lymphatic system. It is an acetylcholinesterase inhibitor, which means that it is good for those with Alzheimer's or Parkinson's diseases. It is the primary herb used for bipolar disorder and schizophrenia. It enhances memory and right brain function. Alcoholics need this herb to repair their brain function after they stop drinking. This herb is a secondary herb to fight tumor formation. It you suffer from brain tumors, it may help to take ashwagandha with bacopa on a nightly basis. The prevention of more tumor formation will allow your brain to repair and your memory to improve. You also will need to take alpha lipoic acid in very high doses to turbo-charge this action. Ashwagandha can help memory loss associated with Parkinson's, Alzheimer's, dementia, depression, anxiety, insomnia, alcoholism, bipolar disorder, schizophrenia, and MS. This adaptogen can increase the life and number of neurons or brain cells in your brain.

> ### Ginger

Ginger is an herb that is a stimulant and is thermogenic in nature. It increases brain circulation and crosses the blood-brain barrier. It increases brain metabolism and may increase the need for vitamins and cofactors in the diet. This herb seems to affect glucose metabolism in a positive way. It can help those with vertigo; it should be tried in tea form as a drink several times a day for this problem. This also may improve the memory of an Alzheimer's patient. This is a great way for older patients with slow metabolism to increase their overall metabolism and brain function. It does increase the energy produced by the brain cells.

➤ Green tea

Green tea is the number two memory enhancer and is widely available around the world. It helps reduce stress and anxiety. Green tea is often available with other ingredients added to the tea bags. It is my recommendation to get the product that you like the best and the improved taste will inspire you to drink more of this health beverage. The green tea liquid extract can allow you to have the benefit of drinking seven to twenty-five cups a day by adding a full dropper into a glass of water. Green tea reduces free radicals and is an antioxidant. It interferes with viral replication in the brain. It can slow the destructive forces caused by virus like herpes, HIV, CMV, HPV, hepatitis, or rotovirus and it can reverse the damage caused by these viruses for some people. It can be useful in managing and treating migraine headaches. Many brain problems are caused by bacteria and virus getting into the bloodstream and crossing into brain. When they have not been diagnosed and treated, they can develop into major brain diseases. MS and ALS are caused by viruses.

Green tea is a stimulant and relaxant at the same time. These properties are usually found in adaptogens. This herb is extremely important in brain function because it can chelate excess iron. It enhances learning ability and is the number-two anti-aging herb of all time. It is the most affordable way to enhance brain health. It is antibacterial, antiviral, anti-fungal, and crosses the blood brain barrier. It helps prevent cancer, and for this reason it should be included in most people's diets.

Other beneficial herbs to enhance brain function include:

➤ Mucuna pruriens

➤ Yohimbe

➤ Bilberry

➤ Fo-ti

➤ Kelp

➤ Shu di huang

➤ Rosemary

➤ Sophora

- ➤ Schizandra berry
- ➤ Polygonatum silibicum root
- ➤ Red panax ginseng
- ➤ Jyotishmati, or Celastrus panniculats
- ➤ Huperzine A
- ➤ Galantamine
- ➤ Rehmannia
- ➤ Betony
- ➤ Peppermint
- ➤ Morning glory (Evolvulus alsinoides)

Bio-Energetic Synchronization Technique (BEST)

Bio-Energetic Synchronization Technique (BEST) is a neurological refining technique developed by Dr. M. T. Morter Jr., a chiropractor in Arkansas. BEST is a non-forceful, energy-balancing, hands-on procedure used to help reestablish the full healing potential of the body. BEST has been researched at major universities, including the University of California, and taught in several chiropractic colleges and in professional continuing education seminars.

Its principles acknowledge the concept of interference that we create with our conscious mind. This interference causes imbalance in the autonomic nervous system, leading to exhaustion of our organ systems over time. BEST uses gentle touch to resynchronize misaligned body magnetic fields. It may be combined with other modalities, depending upon the physical and mental state of the patient.

BEST is based on the scientific principle of bio-magnetic fields. It utilizes light pressure contacts on the surface of the body to address parasympathetic and sympathetic imbalances. When expressed in the intrinsic muscles of the spine as a chiropractic subluxation, pinched nerve, or muscle spasm, imbalances can lead to symptoms of discomfort and loss of body functions. Brain function is often impaired by misaligned spinal columns, and this reduces available central nervous system signals throughout the body and in the brain. This type of approach can be astounding for those unfamiliar with it.

Physical BEST procedure offers a non-forceful way to release patterns of stress and discomfort that create acute pain and chronic conditions. It is administered with the patient in the prone position, utilizing the prone leg check to evaluate the length of both legs to see if one is shorter, palpating the spinal muscles, and subsequently holding pressure points along the spine, sacrum, and skull. When muscles are balanced and the updated pattern restored, spinal muscle spasm, vertebral subluxation, and nerve pressure are removed. The body can heal itself if just given the opportunity finding the power within yourself and using it to raise your brain power and clear your thinking.

Emotional BEST utilizes advanced technology developed to update higher brain interference from expression in the physical body. When any emotion worry, guilt, fear, or judgment—becomes the primary factor in our memory patterns, interference with the divine plan for our perfect health and wellness becomes the norm. This interference, formulated by conscious thought, which in turn becomes a pattern, prevents the true expression of our physical bodies' healing capability. Emotional BEST is an advanced procedure to help identify this emotional pattern, update the interference, and then allow the body to function, based on current situations rather than past experiences. The core of BEST technology results in health and wellness. This procedure can be utilized by both practitioners and patients, depending on their level of expertise. It usually takes between five and fifteen minutes to complete. More on this technique can be found on Dr. Morter's website at www.morter.com.

Intravenous Nutritional Therapy

The Myers Cocktail is an intravenous therapy that consists of mixing vitamins, minerals, amino acids, and other nutrients. It can be very useful in treating autoimmune diseases, chronic illness, viral infections, brain illness, diabetes, or digestive problems where oral nutrients are not being absorbed. When nutrients are given intravenously, your digestive system is bypassed, and a much higher level of nutrition can be delivered directly to your cells via the bloodstream. Vitamin B12 and other B vitamins in IV offer almost immediate support to your brain metabolism and speed waste removal from your neurons.

The Myers Cocktail improves almost all digestive symptoms, including bloating, diarrhea, food allergies, irritable bowel syndrome, colitis, ulcers, and Crohn's disease. Impaired digestion issues frequently affect clear thinking and your brain. The Myers Cocktail intravenous therapy improves the body's ability to make energy and increases cellular function. You may feel a warm sensation while the IV is administered.

The Myers Cocktail IV therapy may be helpful for impaired brain issues, concentration problems, learning challenges, and memory loss due to chronic or acute conditions like mental fatigue, diabetes, herpes, HIV, CMV, HPV, hepatitis, PTSD, fatigue, fibromyalgia, depression, bacterial or viral infection, asthma, cardiac pain, congestive heart failure, palpitations, migraine headaches, cardiovascular disease, respiratory problems, seasonal allergies, hives, hyperthyroidism, and hormone problems. Severe health concerns increase the cellular need for vitamins, minerals, cofactors, trace mineral salts, amino acids, and protein levels.

Emotional Component of IQ and Brain Function

Emotional blockage can impair brain focus and ability to function. Bach Flower Remedies can be used successfully to reduce and dissipate emotional trauma, stress, and blockages connected to IQ. This is especially true for children and teenagers. As the emotions are processed, the brain will perform at a higher level. Bach Flower Remedies are a great option for children due to their toxic-free nature.

Bach Flower Remedies by Dr. Bach, who developed thirty-eight different flower essences or remedies, remain popular and available in many parts of the world. Australian Bush Flower Essences and California Essences are available in addition to the original Bach remedies. Flower remedies are an integral part of holistic medicine.

Music Therapy

Music therapy, Acutonics (harmonic sound and vibrational healing), singing, and Tibetan singing bowls are simpler versions of the concept of using music or sound vibrations to heal stress, anxiety, or more serious problems. A relaxed brain retains information better and has a better functioning memory. Learning and IQ can be enhanced. The Hemi-Sync method is a more sophisticated version of vibrational sound therapy. The brain can be enhanced by auditory therapy. The sounds are played on a CD and listened to with headphones. The brain-wave activity is altered by the sound vibration as it is heard. There are several types of brain waves, and your brain may not experience proper brain-wave activity. This adjusts the brainwave activity for higher learning and concentration.

Hemi-Sync works to entrain the brain into the proper brain-wave activity for optimal brain function and memory. Vibrational energy healing is based on the tenet that disease stems from a lack of proper resonance. Music therapy and sound therapy have many successful results.

Health will return when cells are put into vibrational balance. It seems that music therapy may be a way to influence and change neurotransmitter levels. Classical music and baroque music are the best music for balancing the brain. Music therapy with a harp is very good. Classical music has long been associated with high IQ levels in children. Enroll your child in band or piano lessons for higher IQ levels. Ages three to seven is the age range that has great outcomes. Suzuki music lessons are a wonderful way to proceed for extremely young children.

Eye Movement Desensitization and Reprocessing (EMDR)

Eye movement desensitization and reprocessing (EMDR) may be promising. EMDR has reportedly brought dramatic improvement to many of those treated, and it has become standard treatment in some veterans hospitals. The patient visualizes a distressing image from the traumatic event while tracking two fingers the therapist moves quickly back and forth across his line of vision. After each set of movements, the patient reports any new feelings or forgotten memories he may have. The therapist then repeats the procedure. A session lasts about sixty to ninety minutes and is repeated as often as needed. Some patients report that EMDR accomplishes more in one session than conventional counseling has managed in years.

Increasing Neural Stem Cells

Patent US7393830 was issued in July 2008 and discusses increasing neural stem cells with the hormone prolactin. If this is true, vitex (chasteberry or Agnus castus) should be taken to alter prolactin levels. Vitex is an adaptogenic herb that can balance the hormones. It can increase or decrease the level of prolactin. If you have low prolactin, supplementation can assist the anterior lobe of the pituitary gland to increase production of prolactin.

Genetic research is focusing on altering intelligence with gene therapy. Intelligence is associated with the X chromosome, and there are recent discoveries that correlate certain diseases to intelligence. Myopia or nearsightedness is one of the positive genetic correlations. It is unknown if in genetic correlations that altering one side symptom changes other genetically correlated issues like myopia. If myopia is linked with high IQ's, would the techniques that repair the DNA to restore eye sight also lower IQ over time?

Chinese Herbal Formulas

There are many problems related to memory, brain fog, concentration and intelligence. TCM memory-enhancing formulas are often found to be anti-aging in nature. They can increase the life of neurons and increase information flow from right to the left hemisphere of the brain. In Oriental medicine, these problems are usually connected with blood deficiency, kidney yang, kidney essence deficiency, qi deficiency, and others. The following Chinese herbal formulas can increase memory, intelligence, concentration, clarity, and/or focus:

Gui Pi Wan improves memory.

Huan Shao Dan Wan improves memory.

Ren Shen Shou Wu Pian can improve memory and add about three to twelve IQ points.

Bu Nao Pian is a general brain tonic that tonifies and increases brain circulation.

Immortal Qi Patent Formula or Bu Zhong Yi Qi Tang He Sheng Mai San Jia Jian by Blue Poppy increases qi and yin to improve memory and intelligence and is anti-aging.

Lu Wei Di Huang Tang enhances cognitive ability and increases the speed at which information can be processed. It can increase the speed at which tests can be taken.[1]

Orthomolecular Medicine

The following are brain enhancing amino acid and nutritional supplements to improve memory, concentration, and intelligence:

➢ Acetyl-L-Carnitine

Carnitine helps bring molecules from the body's fat stores to cells as energy to burn. It moves fatty acids through cellular membranes and cytosol into cells' mitochondria, where the fats undergo oxidation to produce ATP and increase cellular energy. Acetyl-L-carnitine influences the regulation of the hormone pregnenolone produced by the adrenal gland. Pregnenolone deficiency is associated with low energy and extreme fatigue. Carnitine is found primarily in meat and dairy foods. Carnitine increases IQ by increasing the energy level of the neuron, which improves memory and allows better storage of memory. Concentration skills are improved along with mental focus.

➢ DL-Phenylalanine

DL-phenylalanine is an amino acid that is a precursor for tyrosine. It affects the levels of dopamine, norepinephrine, noradrenaline, and adrenaline. It is useful in treating alcoholism, ADHD, Parkinson's, and depression. It is useful in the area of memory loss related to hormone deficiencies, depression, and neurotransmitter imbalances. It can also increase attention span and concentration.

➢ GABA

GABA is an amino acid used for depression, insomnia, and anxiety. It may be very effective for those people who cannot use antidepressants due to side effects. Depression is usually associated with memory loss, and the deeper depressions cause more serious memory loss.

GABA is an amino acid that is a calming neurotransmitter. It is usually deficient in those with depression and anxiety. People with high levels of anxiety have difficulty retaining information and learning. People with inadequate sleep also have difficult times with memory, learning, concentration, and mental sharpness. GABA may also be useful in treating OCD and insomnia. Using GABA for addiction issues should be a long-term strategy. This supplement should be taken for two to five years. Treating addiction issues with amino acid therapy requires a long-term commitment. GABA is not effective in treating severe depression or bipolar disorder.

> ➤ DMAE

DMAE, or dimethylaminoethanol, is stimulant substance found in sardines and anchovies. It was made into a drug found in Europe that is sold under the name Deaner. It has the ability to function very similar to a hormone in the brain. It helps brain function in those over forty. It is similar to choline. DMAE accelerates the speed of mental processing of information. It improves mental alertness, concentration, and clarity of thinking. It helps the brain by addressing behavioral problems associated with ADD and ADHD in men and increases attention span. It can improve motor coordination and compulsive disorders. It may help those with antisocial or behavioral problems.

DMAE can increase IQ, eliminate morning brain fog, increase attention, reduce irritability, and reduce chronic fatigue. This substance improves the way the brain uses essential fatty acids as we age. It can help with movement and motor coordination disorders like Parkinson's. DMAE also can prevent "liver spots" on the hands as we age. It can be used to treat schizophrenia on a long-term basis.

> ➤ L-Tyrosine

Tyrosine is a nonessential amino acid made from phenylalanine. It is a precursor for making brain neurotransmitters. It is turned into epinephrine, dopamine, and norepinephrine. Tyrosine supplementation helps the body adapt to stress-induced memory loss. It can increase neuron communication and improve mood. Tyrosine helps regulate hormones, including adrenal, thyroid, and pituitary hormones.

Tyrosine can be useful in helping those with ADD and ADHD increase mental alertness and concentration. It may be useful in enhancing brain function for those with schizophrenia. It also may help with erectile dysfunction and chronic fatigue. Patients with hypothyroid disease may have a deficiency of tyrosine and improve upon taking this supplement. It can reverse memory loss.

> ➤ Pregnenolone

Pregnenolone is a potent memory enhancer. It is a hormone involved in cognitive function and memory. It is produced by the adrenal glands, gonads, and central nervous system. This hormone improves brain function and delays or prevents the collapse of neurotransmitters during periods of extreme trauma or stress. It is a neuroprotector. Under the right circumstances, pregnenolone can increase the stimulate rate of neurons when combined with other brain supplements. It can function as an activator for alpha lipoic acid, vitamin C, and glutathione. It increases the production of brain cells. It also reduces anxiety, depression, and stress. It increases the amount of available acetylcholine in the brain. It can increase available serotonin and dopamine levels, depending on the patient.

➢ Alpha Lipoic Acid

This cofactor is an antioxidant that restores the function of nerves and protects brain cells from infections and aging. It slows the formation of free radicals in the body and brain and improves cognitive function. It can increase brain alertness and concentration for those with dementia or diabetes. It helps chelate heavy minerals when taken on a daily basis. This is extremely important for brain function for all people with nerve damage or any type illness that attacks the nervous system.

➢ Melatonin

Melatonin is a hormone produced in the brain by the pineal gland from the amino acid tryptophan. It is available as a nutritional supplement. Melatonin is stimulated by darkness and suppressed by light and is affected by the circadian rhythm. It regulates diverse body functions. It can enhance moods and improve concentration. It increases brain functioning with its ability to enhance immune function and increase the brain circulation. It helps restore the brain for those with addiction issues after the withdrawal programs have been completed; it should be taken as a supplement during the withdrawal programs.

➢ Lithium Orotate

Lithium orotate is a trace mineral salt found in RNA and DNA. It can repair damaged nerves. Lithium orotate travels inside the brain to stabilize many of the chemical activities of the neurons and protects brain cells in the hippocampus, striatum, and frontal cortex of the brain. It helps stimulate the growth of new neurons. Any substance that helps grow brain cells can increase IQ. It is especially true for a patient who has been recently diagnosed with a brain disease in the early stage.

➢ CoQ10

Coenzyme Q10 is a ubiquinone. It is a cofactor in energy production and is a coenzyme used in energy production by the mitochondria. CoQ10 affects many neurological functions. It is best taken with food that contains some type of lipid or fat. It is cytoprotective, neuroprotective, and active in the cortex area of the brain. It enhances and protects the immune function. It helps prevent dementia and memory loss. It prevents headaches. It helps the brain fight infection and repair accelerated aging. It slows the decline of the brain.

> Phosphatidylserine (PS)

Phosphatidylserine, or PS, is a phospholipid. It contains both amino acids and essential acids and is a major find in anti-aging brain medicine. It is often made from soy. It can reverse brain aging from nine to twelve years when taken on a long-term regular basis. It is useful for prevention of memory loss and increasing concentration and attention span. This is specifically for memory-related brain problems.

PS helps those with OCD, ADD, ADHD, depression, stress, anxiety, and bipolar disorder. It can be given to children. It helps the brain deal with stress and anxiety. It improves your brain's ability to store and process information. It can be taken without a prescription and found in your health food store.

> DHEA

DHEA is a natural hormone precursor to estrogen and androgen produced from cholesterol in the gonads, adipose tissue, brain, and the skin. Your body's own DHEA levels may be reduced by taking insulin, corticosteroids, opiates, or danazol. It affects the cortex of the brain. DHEA can lower the levels of interleukin-6. DHEA acts as an anti-inflammatory and immune enhancer. DHEA may be reduced by alcohol and drug abuse, severe depression, stress, insomnia, and menopause. It can improve mood and prevent anxiety and stress. It reduces inflammation in the brain and is an antioxidant. It protects the brain and protects the anterior cingulate cortex of the brain. It increases hippocampal activity under nonstressful conditions, which can directly affect IQ. Thin people will often need or can be helped by a DHEA supplement. Anyone with a wasting syndrome, like HIV or cancer, may want to consider a high-quality supplement.

> B12

Vitamin B12 has the ability to enhance brain function in many ways, including preventing dementia and improving memory loss. It improves concentration problems and helps the brain prevent psychological problems. It helps prevent depression. Patients who are diabetic require higher levels of this vitamin in order to protect their nerves and brain from the inflammation caused by the disease.

> Choline

CDP-choline is a form of choline and cytidine. Choline is a precursor to the phosphatidylcholine. It is used in the structure and function of cells. It is a precursor to acetylcholine. CDP-choline can affect many neurological functions. It is a cognitive enhancer and helps support the brain as it matures. It prevents memory loss in most people. It is cytoprotective, neuroprotective, and is active in the temporal area of the brain. It is an antioxidant.

> Piracetam

Piracetam has the ability to transform brain function and repair brain function. It increases the transfer of information between the left and bright brain. People with brain diseases do not always have a good information-transfer skills. This increases cholinergic receptors in the brain. It is able to restore cell membrane fluidity and increase brain circulation. It protects the brain and is a memory enhancer. It can reverse cognitive impairment. It is a great product for those suffering from amnesia associated with brain trauma. It helps depression, anxiety, neurosis, and stress. This may be used to slow the progression of Alzheimer's and reverse early dementia when used along with acupuncture.

> Picamilon

Picamilon is made by combining niacin with GABA. The medical action of picamilon exceeds the combined effects of GABA and niacin. It has the effect of a tranquilizer for many people. It reduces stress while increasing circulation in the brain. It reduces depression, neurosis, and emotional stress. This action allows a higher-functioning level in the brain. It may be able to restore some brain damage. It helps restore brain function in alcoholics during and after alcohol withdrawal and may help the brain regain some function after damage from cocaine.

> Black Cohosh

Black cohosh root is used for brain enhancement and to increase IQ, specifically for people with hormone imbalances of FSH and luteinizing hormone. It binds to the estrogen receptor sites. Menopausal women's brain function can improve with this supplement for about one month. It should be taken for about one year; take it early in the morning on an empty stomach for best results. If there are no results in five weeks, discontinue this supplement and switch to PS. Those with hepatitis, liver cancer, liver disease, or impaired liver function should not take this herb. It is an anti-inflammatory and antibiotic. It improves brain circulation and can prevent insomnia. It also helps migraines. This herb may help improve memory associated to hormone imbalances and may help Alzheimer's and MS patients.

> Theophylline

Theophylline is used to treat those suffering from anxiety or stress. It can relax and calm. It protects, balances, and extends the life of neurons, and this prevents or delays the onset of major brain diseases like dementia, memory loss, cognitive disorders, and autism. Any product that increases the life of brain cells is anti-aging and brain-enhancing.

> DMG

DMG, or dimethylglycine, is a derivative of the amino acid glycine. It is also known as vitamin B15 in Russia. It is used to treat drug addiction, alcoholism, autism, schizophrenia, children with minimal brain damage, senile dementia, and cognitive impairment. It can improve neuron function, sharpen thinking, and improve mental clarity.

Additional options to enhance brain power include:

> Caffeine

> Trimethylglycine (TMG)

> Omega-3 fatty acids

> Lecithin

> Galantamine

> Spirulina

Sex

Research from at the University of Calgary published in 2003 by the *Science Journal* demonstrated that hormones stimulated by sex may cause the production of new brain cells. Sex increases the production of neurotransmitters and hormones, increases the ATP, increases oxygenation, and increases blood circulation, which are key in the formation of neurons. This may extend beyond its effect on stimulating hormones and neurotransmitters to simple stress relief. The reduction of stress reduces inflammation throughout the body and brain. Sex directly increases blood flow throughout the body for a two hour period after sex for added circulatory benefit. The added feelings of closeness after sex often repair damaged relationships and can extend life in married couples.

Emotional Freedom Technique (EFT)

Emotional Freedom Technique, or EFT, is a therapy that excels at treating pain or symptoms related to emotional thoughts, feelings, trauma, or post-traumatic stress disorder (PTSD). Depression can be improved with EFT. This is a fairly inexpensive therapy that can be done with the help of a professional and reinforced by oneself at home. This therapy should be performed initially by an acupuncturist, chiropractor, Orthomolecular Medicine doctor, osteopath, or alternative medicine doctor.

EFT is a relatively new therapy that can benefit many people with disease and emotional trauma. It could alter the electro-magnetic field of the patient. This therapy has not been extensively studied or published, however, and there are not adequate double blind studies on this therapy in America.

EFT uses fingers to perform a tapping motion on acupuncture points along energy meridians established in Traditional Chinese Medicine. This is known as EFT tapping. This process is easy to perform on your own at home after a medical professional shows you the correct way to do the therapy. The points that are tapped must be exactly correct in location. There may be additional points added to your treatment, depending upon your specific injury, disease, or level of emotional distress. This technique usually must be done more than once in order for it to succeed. There are positive and negative affirmations that are stated out loud while the tapping is done.

This therapy can alter your thoughts and feelings. Many diseases can improve and heal when the person changes his or her belief or thought concerning an illness or symptom. Many times, a patient's getting better can be as simple as getting someone to believe he can improve and helping him visualize this change in his life. Tapping may have this ability, along with moving the blocked energy along Chinese energy meridians. There are several energy meridians in the body and they correspond to specific organs.

When the body's energy gets blocked or stuck in a specific organ, like the heart or small intestine, it may impact several organs and energy throughout the entire body. Chinese medicine believes that each energy meridian and organ is connected to emotions directly or indirectly. As energetic blockages are removed and the energy flows freely, the person will improve, and any emotionally caused problems can heal. It is possible for a person to get well in a single treatment, but many people will require several sessions. EFT will not replace hard work in overcoming addictions. It will help in treating addictions and eating disorders. It can be used for healing depression, stress, anxiety, sleep disorders, migraines, seizures, and tics.

Auricular Acupuncture

Auricular acupuncture is often used to increase memory, reduce stress and anxiety, improve concentration, increase focus, and reduce brain fog. The auricular points used for increasing include shen men, subcortex, brain, brain stem, cortex, kidney, spleen, and endocrine. Several sessions will be required, and each session will take from thirty to forty-five minutes. Mourant acupuncture adds gold needles to this treatment, along with a sound meditation of violin, harp, or classical Bach music.

Neurofeedback

Neurofeedback may be used for psychological and stress problems. It can correct many brain imbalances that affect anxiety, stress, anger, depression, chronic stress, memory loss, and concentration problems. Reversing these issues can improve memory and concentration skills. Many people suffer from chronic headaches, migraines, sexual dysfunction, mania, nervous stomach, essential hypertension, brain fog, anger management issues, and fear. These are classic symptoms connected to accelerated aging of brain cells. This is a very good tool for brain issues and may be found at hospitals or psychologists' offices. Ask your doctor for this therapy.

Neurofeedback will improve the transmission of information across the hemispheres and increase neural pathways or strengthen existing neural pathways. This therapy involves sitting in front of a computer screen for about forty-five minutes with headphones on while a program plays on your screen. It may take ten to twenty of these sessions for your memory to significantly increase. If stress reduction is your primary issue, it may happen much more quickly.

Yoga

Yoga is a great way to increase circulation, improve flexibility, reduce stress, balance hormones, restore proper sleep cycles, and improve energy flow. Different types of yoga offer different health benefits. You will have better concentration with balanced hormones and neurotransmitters after a yoga practice of several weeks. Your memory will improve, and your anxiety will subside.

Yoga increases balance, flexibility, and fitness at a gentle pace suitable for almost everyone. People of all ages and levels of fitness can do yoga. Discuss all health problems with the yoga instructor prior to class so you can be guided in which postures need to be avoided for specific health concerns.

Yoga is a great way to detoxify, increase flexibility, balance hormones, and increase metabolism. It also is an amazing tool for athletic people for cross-training or preventing injury.

Speed Learning

Speed Learning is a technique developed by Professor Lozanov and was distributed in the 1970s by Ostrander and Schroeder. This was an experiment that was very successful. This technique will change the lives of all it touches.

The version in my class was put on a projector screen at the front of the class. This technology can more than double your ability to learn math, language, and memory skills. This therapy may also extend to improving the brain's ability to learn a second language more quickly. This technique can help students get acceptance into college and university. It can improve grades to help with university scholarships. It does require some adult supervision for best results.

This technique has been changed since the early seventies and now includes rhythms and frequencies. The summary of their experiments can be found in the book *Superlearning*. This previously very expensive technology is now available on a CD at an inexpensive cost of $19.95 plus tax and shipping at the website.

Good diagnostic testing is the key to the best medicine, along with selecting the best doctor. It is very difficult for those with three or more diseases to manage their medical treatment for the best and most cost effective outcome. The use of medical specialists makes it difficult for those with more than one disease. Choose a doctor whose background is advanced enough to outline the extensive healthcare issues for each of your diseases. It is important to understand which of your diseases is the primary issue and select your medical treatments accordingly. Attempt to understand the root cause of the illnesses and proceed carefully. Choose your treatments, and take good notes to monitor the success of every therapy or herb.

You can find the products and services mentioned in this book, including links to doctors who specialize in the forms of medicine discussed, by visiting http://QuantumBrainHealing.com. Stay tuned for my next book, *Quantum Orthomolecular Medicine*. It will offer new ideas and ways to stay trim and young.[i]

Made in the USA
Lexington, KY
03 May 2014